UNHUNCHED

DISCOVER WELLNESS THROUGH POSTURE

UNHUNCHED

DISCOVER WELLNESS
THROUGH POSTURE

AESHA TAHIR

ILLUSTRATED BY SHAWN LIN

NEW DEGREE PRESS

COPYRIGHT © 2023 AESHA TAHIR

UNHUNCHED

DISCOVER WELLNESS THROUGH POSTURE

ISBN 979-8-88926-926-7 *Paperback*

ISBN 979-8-88926-969-4 *Ebook*

We are all sculptors and painters, and our material is our own flesh and blood and bones.

—HENRY DAVID THOREAU

Table of Contents

Introduction
Caveperson's
Wellness Guide

———

I woke up to a burning pain going down my left leg, accompanied by an unsettling numbness in my foot. It was the strangest sensation.

As I attempted to stand up, struggling to get out of bed, another jolt of radiating pain like an electric current passed through my leg. My mind raced through different possibilities, like a computer program's code running through all the possible outcomes for the user input. I feared I was having a stroke, which, given my family's history of cardiovascular disease, was a certain possibility.

After remaining calm and driving myself to the ER, the physician diagnosed me with sciatica and attributed it to weak core muscles and a sedentary lifestyle. He explained, "Your lower back vertebrae on the left hip are putting pressure on your sciatic nerve."

That visit to the ER marked the start of a three-year search for lower back pain relief. Exploring different solutions, I learned I was neglecting the muscles necessary to maintain a good posture, and sitting hunched over created muscle imbalances. Later, my pain started dissipating when I temporarily stepped away from my work because of motherhood and became more active.

I started looking into our work habits and posture. I knew there was more to postural health than what's already commonly known. Indeed, someone has studied it and would know much more about how it affects our health.

I found a heap of scientific literature, ranging from the survival advantage of unhunched posture to emotional empowerment gained through posture. Through extensive reading and research, I uncovered the mystery of optimal posture and started implementing positive posture habits into my life. As I shared my story with friends and family, they also wanted to learn these habits. That started my professional journey in the health and wellness industry. I began helping busy office workers like me live a pain-free and healthy life by incorporating small habits into their day.

If your work requires a lot of screen time and you spend the majority of your day sitting down, then perhaps you're no stranger to pain. You probably want to get active and find a solution to your pain, but you don't know how to build time into your already overbooked schedule. If nothing else, you just want to overcome the stiffness and tension you feel at the end of the long workday. You're not alone. Over my career, I've helped many people who've shared similar frustrations. That was the case for Karen, who came to see me for neck stiffness.

She told me about what had happened to her, saying, "It was a mistake. I'd only swum four strokes when I turned my head to breathe and felt a sudden sharp pain. It made me feel very sick."

Since that swim in December 2020, Karen has been experiencing episodic, intense headaches. She visited many doctors about this concern, and they concluded it wasn't a neurologic issue. It was a muscular issue. Her neck and shoulder muscles were strained. They recommended improving her desk posture and sedentary behavior.

As an IT specialist for a major insurance company, Karen's long work hours stressed her out. Most days, she worked an average of twelve hours sitting in the same spot from dawn to dusk. Two weeks prior, she had decided to start swimming after work, having enjoyed it as a high school and college athlete. Unfortunately, this decision resulted in a neck injury.

Upon evaluation, I found the cause of her neck injury was sitting with a slumped posture and a forward head position to get a better view of the computer screen. Sitting in a slumped position with a computer monitor that is too low puts extra pressure on the neck, leading to headaches. "I know I am in front of the computer many hours each day, but I never thought it could be so detrimental to my health," she said, staring at me in disbelief.

Unfortunately, Karen's situation is not unique. Poor posture and musculoskeletal issues are becoming increasingly common due to our sedentary lifestyle. This behavior is at an all-time high for office workers. Researchers found that office workers spend 75 percent of their waking hours sitting down (Hazlegreaves 2019), which amounts to twelve hours of sitting daily.

Like many professionals, Karen wasn't aware of her body position because she was so engrossed in her work. However, this lack of awareness can have long-term implications. Because of the modern work culture's obsession with efficiency and multitasking, our awareness of the environment and body has reduced. We work on autopilot, like the computer programs we work with (APA 2006).

How long can our bodies take this type of strain? The answer is not for too long. In Karen's case, it was neck pain. Karen's already tight and aching muscles couldn't handle additional pressure from the swim, which led to severe neck pain and headaches. For many office workers, the overtaxing of muscles leads to poor sleep, low confidence, ineffective communication, cardiovascular diseases, metabolic conditions like diabetes, and psychological disorders like anxiety and depression.

So, is all the blame on Karen for being a committed employee and athlete? No, it's not. Like any other behavior, our environment plays a key role in our posture. Our body naturally adjusts to our surroundings to fight gravity. It tries to balance us no matter what, even if that means sacrificing optimal alignment as we sit at work.

To understand the prevalence of musculoskeletal issues today, we will take a walk through history. It took millions of years for our prehistoric human ancestors to develop this unhunched posture to fight the gravitational pull. The unhunched posture provided them with a survival advantage. Over time they evolved into extremely active, upright species that spread globally.

Our ancestors protected their health for years while hunting, building tools, and adopting agriculture. Even today, back, neck, and shoulder pain are unheard of in some indigenous tribes. Members of these tribes live long, functional, and pain-free lives. This book will challenge your beliefs about old age and posture. You will learn about the lifestyles of those tribes and how you can apply their wisdom to your busy lives. You will also learn many ways to assess your posture.

Today, we are hunched over and sedentary. Our work ecosystem is no longer in sync with our bodies. Technology is a new constant in our lives, and it comes with many conveniences. However, the effects of technology go beyond only convenience.

It's not just Karen who suffers from pain. Lower back pain is the leading cause of disability globally (Health Policy Institute 2019). Fifty percent of all working Americans, the equivalent of eighty million people, experience back pain annually. Our postural health has financial consequences too. Lower back pain alone is a $50 billion problem, not including lost wages and decreased productivity (American Chiropractic Association, 2020). Why wouldn't it be a problem? According to the American Heart Association, sedentary jobs have increased by 83 percent since 1950.

In today's digital age, many working professionals consistently look down at their screens, sinking into their chairs for hours on end. Our hunched posture in front of computers is far from natural. The body of a modern human is working against its evolutionary physiology. That's why I wrote this book. I wrote it to give people like Karen and you a road map to discover wellness. It provides a framework in synergy with our evolutionary physiology and technological advances to protect our health and well-being.

Prior to embarking on my posture journey, I believed posture only affected our skeletal system and supportive structures such as muscles. However, as I dived deeper into the science, I discovered dysfunctional breathing, amplified work stress, and low emotional health impact the stability of our body's structures. Posture isn't just about the alignment of our body. It is about the orientation of our mind and body in this world. This book aims to illustrate the relationship between your posture, pain, breathing, work stress, and leadership prowess. You'll find many practical posture tips to let you step into greatness and empower you beyond a pain-free life.

Our desk posture isn't limited to how we sit or stand in a static position. It also comes along with us when we move. It becomes the new normal for our bodies, and our nervous system stops adapting to other recruitment patterns, which like in Karen's case, causes muscle strain, inflammation, and nerve compression.

Through my work with clients like Karen, I realized how widespread the posture health issue is. The World Health Organization estimates 3.2 million premature deaths yearly due to a sedentary lifestyle. That makes hunched-over, sedentary living the fourth largest cause of death globally (World Health Organization 2022).

Many clients come to me without understanding how severely their posture has deteriorated. They can't lift their arms beyond chest height. Some have accepted their fate of living with pain. When I introduce them to my BRACE posture correction model, they finally find the relief they were looking for. The BRACE model stands for breath, relaxation, activity, and corrective exercise. This book contains practical exercises that are field-oriented and backed by research. The best part is you can readily use this model in any setting without a significant investment of equipment or time.

My clients are the primary inspiration for this book. By sharing their stories, I hope to demonstrate the impact of hunched-over sitting on your health. Although there is no such thing as a perfect posture, achieving good health through natural posture is possible and should be the goal. You'll see the term deskbound professionals used in this book often. This term comes from Dr. Kelly Starrett's book, *Deskbound*, which served as an inspiration for this book. In addition, you'll find the stories of some elite athletes and how they have tapped into human potential by using their posture to elevate their performance.

The *Guardian*'s headline on August 16th, 2009, read, "Usain Bolt breaks world record in a time of 9.58 sec to win 100 meters gold in Berlin." Today, ask any kid on the block: they know Usain Bolt is the fastest man to tread this earth. What the kids don't know is that Usain Bolt has scoliosis, a genetic disorder that causes an abnormal sideways curve of the spine (AANS 2009).

"When I was younger, it wasn't really a problem. But you grow, and it gets worse. My spine is really curved bad," says Bolt in an ESPN magazine interview (Howard 2011). Scoliosis most often limits people's lives, with the only hope being spinal surgery to possibly cure it. It didn't limit Bolt. He used the knowledge of his condition as a power. "The early part of my career, when we didn't really know much about it, it really hampered me because I got injured every year," he shares. "I keep my core and back strong. The scoliosis doesn't really bother me."

If the fastest man on earth with a postural genetic anomaly can break world records by changing his training style, then so can you. His example demonstrates how we can use corrective exercise to find better health and optimal pain-free movement.

You're holding a practical wellness guide for modern-day humans, evolved from Stone Age cave dwellers, who sit in front of computers and wish to lead healthier lives. By choosing to read this book, you have already taken the initial step toward reprogramming your brain and body. The process of change has started. So, come along, sit tall, soften your shoulders, and take a deep breath with me as we discover wellness through posture.

PART 1

EVOLUTION AND HISTORY

CHAPTER 1

Pull of Posture

After scoring the tying goal for his team in the 2006 FIFA World Cup, Marco curled up in disbelief with his feet under him and his head on the turf. The crowd cheered as the number 23 on his blue soccer jersey flashed across TV screens around the world. He lifted his head moments later, tears streaming down his face as the cameras zoomed in on his emotions.

Through hours of practice, Marco Materazzi honed his soccer skills, specifically perfecting his body position to land the ball in the net. The key was learning to transfer his momentum to the ball by leaning forward and dropping his center of gravity, which allowed him to overcome gravity and guide the ball into the opponent's net while airborne.

Like Marco, we've all felt the effects of gravitational pull and how we adjust our center of gravity while riding our bikes uphill and carrying our backpacks.

This force is also responsible for aligning our bodies in a symmetrical posture. Gravity is a force always acting on our body, and how our body resists gravity significantly impacts our posture and spine health.

WHAT IS POSTURE?

"Sit up straight." You might have heard this advice from your mother or grandma. She might be more concerned about your appearance than the gravitational forces. But it's worth noting that your grandma understood the benefits of proper posture—something our generation is losing fast.

Posture is the way we stand, sit, lie down, and move. The alignment of our shoulders, neck, back, hips, and the three curves of the spine help our body stay balanced while we hold our posture. In our natural alignment, our skeleton can resist the forces of gravity with the least stress and pressure on the body's supportive structures, like our muscles and ligaments.

There is a particular point in our bodies where the forces of gravity converge. The center of gravity (COG) is the point at which the upper body and lower body's weight are balanced. For most of us, this is just below our naval, halfway between the belly and lower back in a standing position. It is here that the forces of gravity concentrate on our body. Our center of gravity moves with the shift in our posture. We watch dancers and tight-rope walkers in amazement as they move their center of gravity outside their bodies in fascinating ways and remain balanced.

You've moved your center of gravity outside your body many times by hinging at your waist to bend over and pick up your Amazon delivery. In the same way, when you sit at your office desk hunched over, your center of gravity moves forward.

Florence Kendall was a pioneer in the field of physical therapy and posture evaluation and defined posture in relation to gravitational pull. Through her work, she found our body faces the least stress from gravitational pull when all body parts stack effortlessly along an imaginary line. Kendall writes, "[Posture is] a vertical line that intersects the center of gravity and specific body landmarks, namely, the ear, shoulder, hip, knee, and ankle in a lateral position" (Kendall 2010). Thus, the center of gravity defines our natural posture.

Good Posture When Standing

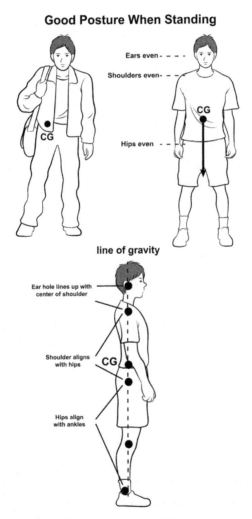

Caption: Center of Gravity and Line of Gravity

GRAVITY'S CONTRIBUTION TO POSTURE

The force of gravity advances the degeneration of bones and joints if our skeletal muscles deviate from this imaginary postural line. If the body hinges forward, as office workers often do, the pull of gravity is exaggerated on our bones, muscles, and joints.

When the gravitational load on our skeletal system increases, our muscles tense up and the structure of our bones slowly starts deteriorating. Over time the bones grow bone spurs to accommodate the load, resulting in a heightened risk of injury and pain at the joint. The pressure from gravity also compresses our spine, resulting in lower back pain and loss of height with age. The increased gravitational pull from slumping forward leads to even further degeneration of the bones. That's how a poor posture, over the career span, can cause our body to wear out in ways it normally wouldn't if it was in its natural alignment.

CARRYING THE LOAD

One of the other ways the impact of gravitational pull on our body increases is from carrying heavy bags over our shoulders. Carrying something heavy shifts our center of gravity. A heavy suitcase or backpack can add weight to specific body parts, distorting our posture.

Wearing your office bag over one shoulder causes leaning to the dominant side of the body to offset the extra weight. "Anything with uneven weight distribution will essentially lead to more muscle imbalances as your body compensates for the weight distribution," says Dr. Jonathan Leary, founder of Remedy Place (Flinn 2019). You can develop lower and upper back pain and strain your shoulders and neck because of the weight imbalance. Shoulder bags and cross-body bags are worst for your posture.

There are a few ways to evenly distribute the weight across your body and align your center of gravity.

- Use a small bag pack to carry your work laptop and other items. A smaller bag will keep the load light and distribute the weight evenly over both sides of your body.

- Reorganize your bag at least once a week to eliminate items you don't need anymore. Heavy backpacks lead to postural scoliosis by moving the body forward (Bettany-Saltikov and Cole 2012).

- If carrying a sling bag is your only option, try to shift it from shoulder to shoulder periodically to even out the load.

LET'S LIVE IN ZERO-G

What if we could take the gravitational force away? Unfortunately, the answer isn't to live without it, either. Without gravity, our body goes through many negative physiological changes.

On April 12, 1961, Yuri Gagarin became the first human to experience life without gravity in a controlled environment. Since then, many astronauts have orbited the Earth and other planets without experiencing gravity's weight. But did you know, upon landing, these astronauts are ushered onto stretchers and must receive medical care to readjust their bodies and physiological systems to Earth's gravity?

The lack of G-forces up in space results in severe bone loss, weak muscles, reduced pressure on the spine, and redistribution of blood. In such an environment, the body views muscles as unnecessary, and they start weakening. Our major postural muscles—like the muscles of the calves and spine that maintain our posture—start losing strength in space. During a two-week space flight, muscle mass diminishes by 20 percent (Clément 2005). The explosive strength of these muscles decreases by 50 percent (Seibert 2001). And bone density drops by 12 percent (Shackelford 2008). All these are markers of overall muscle weakening.

Astronauts are healthy, high-performing individuals who live in an atypical environment. It doesn't surprise a movement scientist like me that they have trouble maintaining an upright posture when they return to Earth. But space travel isn't the only environment that can bring on bone and muscle degeneration. Muscle weakness and bone density loss can result from an injured bone that's immobile in a cast or when our work lives demand long sedentary days.

Sedentary work environments that weaken our muscles due to immobility are far from typical for the human body.

Luckily, it's easy to determine whether your posture effectively fights the gravitational pull.

DIAGNOSING YOUR POSTURE

It's time to evaluate your posture to know where to focus more attention. You will conduct a self-postural analysis, which you can perform independently or with a friend to help you.

We will focus on four critical landmarks for determining our posture: ears, shoulders, hip bones, and feet.

Standing as naturally as possible, take a series of photographs, one from the front and one standing sideways. Standing in front of an empty wall works best for these pictures. Once you've taken your photos, assess the following landmarks in the front view.

- Earlobes: Are your earlobes the same height?

- Shoulders: Are both your shoulders in line with each other? Could you draw a straight line between the two ends of your shoulders?

- Hips: Are the tops of your hips leveled horizontally?

- Feet: Are your feet pointing forward and evenly touching the ground on all four sides?

From the side view, make the following assessments.

- Do your earlobes line up with your shoulder?

- Are your shoulders stacked above your hip bones?

- Do your feet line up under your hip bones?

Does your posture align at these landmarks? If it does, you have a natural posture that can optimally fight the gravitational pull. If these landmarks don't align, you can learn what natural posture looks like by taking the wall test.

WALL TEST

- Stand against a wall. Take a few deep breaths and march a few times in place. Your heels should be about six inches away from the wall. The back of your head, shoulder blades, and butt should be touching the wall.

- Keep your feet shoulder-width apart and your neck straight with your gaze forward. Slide your hand behind your lower back, palm flat, toward the wall. Your wrist should barely slide between the wall and your back for a correct spinal alignment. Pass your hand behind your neck and look if you can slide it the same way. Again, your hand should barely pass through.

- Alternatively, you can have a friend measure the distance between the two points (neck and waist) and the wall. You have a natural posture if the space is two inches or less. You have an excessive spinal curve if it's more than two inches.

- To practice your natural posture, tighten your abdominal muscles by pulling them toward your spine and retract your chin to correct the neck posture if the gap is over two inches. Step away from the wall and hold this posture as long as possible. This is your natural body posture.

Wall Test for Posture Diagnosis

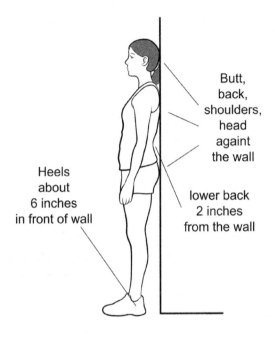

Butt, back, shoulders, head against the wall

Heels about 6 inches in front of wall

lower back 2 inches from the wall

NATURAL POSTURE FOR A BALANCED BODY

When I tell people I am a movement specialist, they tend to become tense and adopt a rigid posture, with their chest lifted, lower back arched, and knees locked. Many individuals aspire to maintain this posture, and I can empathize with their reaction.

When I started my posture journey, I used to force myself into a rigid posture. I would set reminders during the workday to straighten up, but that didn't help. I perpetually hunched over my keyboard. I was about to give up on good posture until my physical therapist explained that a natural posture isn't forced and comes with daily practice of good posture habits.

Now I coach my clients the same way. Standing and moving like a rigid robot is not the answer. Instead, my posture program takes them back to the relaxed and mechanically efficient posture they had as toddlers. The movement is not only pain-free, but also restriction-free.

UPSHOT OF GRAVITY

The upshot of gravity is that it defines our posture. Our natural posture preserves the strength of our muscles and bones. A body aligned vertically with the gravitational line can withstand gravitational pressure. When a person's posture deviates from this straight line, the body exerts additional effort to maintain equilibrium against gravitational forces. Embracing the natural alignment of our skeleton is essential to finding an effortless, fatigue-free posture. It provides the foundation for better movement, shock absorption, pain prevention, and happiness.

Posture Challenge: Try the posture assessment test and the wall test. Increased awareness of how your body reacts to gravitational pull will encourage you to assume your natural posture.

The human musculoskeletal structure emerged because of evolutionary changes in our quadrupedal ancestors' bodies in response to the forces of gravity.

CHAPTER 2

Becoming Unhunched

———

Looking up from his wide-brimmed hat, my toddler said, "Mom, do you think Louis is angry? Is that why he is standing?"

Seeing the excitement and fear in my toddler's eyes reminded me that upright posture is a uniquely human trait. Standing behind the ape enclosure at Philadelphia Zoo, I saw the gorilla striding across the yard with a banana in his hand. I replied, "No, honey, he's trying to get a better look at his little zoo fans like you. He can't see far on four legs." Like my son, we are all fascinated by animals' upright, humanlike stride. I found out Louis the gorilla often walked upright.

Eighteen-year-old Louis became a social media celebrity in 2018 after a zoo volunteer posted a video of him walking like a human on the internet. The video shows this 470-pound silverback gorilla walking upright across the zoo yard, holding two fistfuls of tomatoes.

HUMAN OR APE

"What's unique about him is he doesn't just do it for a couple of steps. He'll walk clear across the yard sometimes," says Michael Stern, the Philadelphia Zoo primate curator, in a WHYY YouTube interview (Fox 2018).

Humans have much in common with other social mammals with grasping hands, bony and enclosed eye sockets, and relatively large brains. These social mammals and humans share a common ancestor. In fact, anthropologists find drawing the line between human and ape fossil records very challenging. All great apes can do many things humans can, like building nests in trees, using tools, and strategically planning their social lives.

"Gorillas and humans are quite similar. We share about 98 percent of our DNA. And that goes down to if you take a close look at their hands, they have fingerprints just like we do," Stern explains. We are functionally close to these mammals too. Stern continues, "All of our internal organs are identical to the point that when we have to do a medical exam on the gorillas, here, we call in human specialists to help us out. We'll have human anesthesiologists and human surgeons. Human OBGYNs are helping us with the females."

Our last common ancestors lived between ten million and seven million years ago (Choi 2017). Shortly after that, our ancestors' species diverged into two separate lineages. One lineage evolved into gorillas and chimpanzees, and the other into early humans or hominids (O'Neil 2012). The earliest hominids started standing straight on two feet in eastern, central, and southern Africa about six million years ago.

Our species' upright bipedal walking is a novelty in the animal kingdom. Humans are the single species out of thousands of mammals and countless animals on this planet that are naturally completely unhunched. Our unhunched posture comes from the copious evolutionary forces on our hominid ancestors' bodies.

DAWN OF UPRIGHT POSTURE

Human anatomy has evolved significantly from those ancestors who walked on all fours, and scientists are studying the evolutionary factors that prompted humans to stand upright and walk on two feet. Evidence from excavated bone fragments, such as skulls, jaws, feet, and pelvic bones, provides the primary basis for this research. Archeologists create partial skeletons and use the DNA from bones to depict the hominids' environment. Understanding the skeletal changes of our ancestors' bodies helps explain what role each body part has in maintaining an upright posture.

Dr. Jan Simek, a paleolithic archaeologist and distinguished professor of science at the University of Tennessee, studies the relationship between the culture and biology of early hominids. He explains to me in our Zoom interview, "When looking at the fossils, the main structural change in hominid anatomy is in the postcranial skeleton [at the bottom of the skull] below the neck and really from the waist down [especially] the relationship between the long bones of the leg and how they articulate at the hip."

He continues, "We see these changes began about six million years ago. We can also see inhabitants of continents were bipedal around three and a half million years ago because we have discovered their footprints." These are the Laetoli footprints, the earliest humanlike footprints found so far, where three people walked together through wet volcanic ash in present-day Tanzania.

Chimpanzees, being quadrupedal, face higher locomotion costs due to limited knee and hip extension. Their hip, thigh, and lower leg bone structure differs from ours. Unlike humans, chimpanzees distribute gravity uniformly across their bodies while walking on all fours. The most crucial transformation in hominid skeletons that gave rise to humans was the evolution of the pelvis to support upright posture, which remains essential for human postural health.

In my graduate Exercise Science program, a great amount of emphasis was placed on the pelvis, a wide dish-shaped bony structure in humans. The long hip bone, also called the femur, inserts into the pelvis like a ball rolls in a cup. The muscles around the hip bone help us maintain equilibrium and stand tall against gravity.

The next question many scientists are trying to answer is why our ancestors evolved to stand unhunched?

THE SURVIVAL ADVANTAGE

Our ancestors found standing straight advantageous for their survival. Changes in their external landscapes encouraged early hominids to move toward warmer climates, where they had to look over the tall grass. "We evolved into upright species because the conditions favored the natural selection of those genes," Dr. Simek explains. "The line of sight becomes a more important characteristic. Our upright posture resulted in protection from the predators that [would] otherwise prey on them out there."

Passing down the upright posture genes to future generations became necessary for survival. After all, natural selection favors the reproduction of offspring with helpful survival traits. Because organisms with beneficial traits leave more offspring, those traits spread widely in the next generation. This way, organisms slowly start adapting to their environment. Standing upright is one such trait.

EVOLUTIONARY FITNESS

Leslea Hlusko, president of the American Association of Biological Anthropologists and researcher at UC Berkley, joined me for a Zoom interview from Burgos, Spain, where she works at the National Research Center on Human Evolution (CENIEH). On the topic of how long this type of adaptation takes, she says, "Thinking about an evolutionary timeframe, we're talking about hundreds and thousands of generations."

All the changes happening during our quadrupedal ancestors' evolution increased the evolutionary fitness of upright humans. "When I look at the primary selective advantage, it has to do with being able to care for more than one young child at a time for our ancestors," says Professor Hlusko. The ability to walk for more extended periods, more efficiently on two legs, in an upright position, and while carrying babies in their hands are some of the ways our unhunched posture increased the evolutionary fitness of our ancestors—all of which helped our species to spread globally.

FUTURE HUMAN EVOLUTION

The pace of human evolution has increased with the advent of agriculture and modern-day cities (Ward 2012). Just like millions of years ago, as our environment changes, we are still adapting and evolving as a species. So, assuming survival amidst future environmental and social conditions, what will our species look like in a millennium?

To answer that question, researchers have collaborated with 3D designers to explore the impact of technology use on posture and speculate on the appearance of future humans. The resulting model, named Mindy, features various anatomical changes due to technological reliance, such as clawlike hands from excessive smartphone use and a permanently bent ninety-degree elbow position from typing (Melore 2022). Mindy's hunched-over posture reflects the position commonly assumed while using tech devices. Additionally, her brain is smaller as future humans will require less thinking to survive.

This study may posit an extreme prediction, and we might challenge it by saying, how can a future human like Mindy result from natural selection? But even if Mindy's exact modeling is debatable, our social and work conditions nevertheless affect our evolutionary fitness in several ways. Take the example of our imbalanced desk posture, which can lead to hereditary chronic diseases like diabetes, heart disease, and hypertension. These diseases create a variation in our genes, which may pass down to future generations.

A hunched posture that puts stress on the body can also directly influence our offspring's health and well-being. "There have been several studies that show when women are under severe stress during pregnancy, the stress affects the metabolic function of a baby and can have a lifelong negative impact on babies' health and well-being," Dr. Hlusko says. "When a baby is in utero, if it's on the path to being a female, we know now that the seven million eggs the female has are already developed while she's still in her mother's uterus. In this way, we can see that grandmother's health and well-being influence how those eggs of her grandchildren will be."

If our future generations inherit musculoskeletal stress and metabolic diseases due to poor posture, then improving our lifestyle to become healthy is vital to preserving our evolutionary fitness and the future of our species.

UPSHOT OF EVOLUTION

The upshot of evolution is that we stood upright and walked on two feet because it provided a survival advantage to our species. Many factors like environmental change, escaping predators, and carrying babies are hypothesized as possible explanations for this shift of our human ancestors to an upright species. Unhunched posture gave our ancestors a survival advantage through better reproductive fitness. To accomplish this, our pelvic region helps us maintain a proper posture.

Posture Challenge: I want to challenge you to spend five minutes daily strengthening your pelvic area or core. Conserving our postural health is one answer to the survival and health of our future generations.

CHAPTER 3

The Ancient Posture

———

As she stood among the weather-worn stone pillars surrounded by grass and beaten brick buildings, she couldn't
help but marvel at the sophistication of this civilization.
However, her thoughts were interrupted by the guide's voice
saying, "At this very spot, Alexander the Great triumphantly
entered the city in 326 BC."

The sixth-grade field trip group immediately stopped
talking. The guide had their full attention now. He continued
explaining how Alexander the Great had invaded the Indus
River Basin. His words painted a vivid picture of the histor-
ical events that happened here several hundred years ago.

Later, inside the museum, he pointed to many faceless
baked statues and stone carvings of yogic figures. As they
continued to move around the exhibits, he stopped at one
and explained, "This is the most ancient seal in the world,
which was found in Harappa, close to the present-day city of
Lahore, Pakistan. It dates to 2500 BC." The sixth-grader was
in awe as she looked at the figure's long spine, bent knees,
legs flat on the ground, and feet touching his hips. The

image is the most ancient known representation of symmetric posture among sculptures. It left her with a renewed appreciation for the region's rich culture and history.

This sixth-grade girl is the descendent of the Indo-European Aryans who settled in the Indus Valley around 2000 BCE. Now, years later, she is connecting her ancestors' ancient movement practices to maintaining good posture and health in the technological age.

I'm that girl!

HUNTER-GATHERERS

Africa is widely known as the original homeland of human beings. About 100,000 years ago, our species began to migrate out of Africa, colonizing the Middle East, South Asia, and Australia (Gugliotta 2008).

As humans started to adapt and exploit the new environments, they learned to consume new foods and explore different lifestyles. Most early human tribes were nomadic, carrying only the most essential belongings. Eventually, these tribes started cultivating crops along the river basins, leading to the development of nascent agricultural communities. Evidence from ancient cave art shows these communities began developing tools to domesticate animals and preserve crops.

While the development of agriculture provided many benefits, it also had some adverse health effects. The relatively more sedentary lifestyle from farming gave rise to an increased rate of arthritis and anemia compared to nomadic hunter-gatherer forebears. But these early civilizations also recognized the benefits of prioritizing health by incorporating exercise and movement into their lifestyle. This allowed them to maintain their well-being and physical health as their lifestyles evolved.

SANCTUARY IN CYPRUS

Located right at the intersection of Africa, Asia, and Europe, Cyprus is a unique island and home to archeological findings from the Stone Age. The Cyprus exhibit at Stockholm's Medelhavsmuseet, the Museum of the Mediterranean and Near East, shows agricultural communities' early lifestyle.

Upon entering the museum building, I was enthralled by some small exhibits that displayed clay pots from ancient Cypriot civilizations. I started my tour on the main floor gallery with an audio guide informing me, "Reputed for its masses of terracotta votive statuary, [the village of] Ayia Irini has produced one the richest corpora of figures and figurines ever to have been excavated in the ancient Mediterranean."

As I continued through the museum, my jaw dropped at the sight of nearly a thousand terracotta figures. These figures date back to Middle Archaic Period, around 8,000 years ago (Osteen, Ledbetter, and Elliott 2017). What struck me most about the sculptures was their straight backs, open chests, broad shoulders, and thin waistlines—all of which highlight their overall unhunched postures.

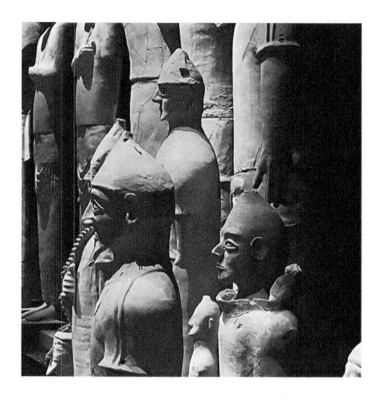

Caption: Terracotta Figures from Cyprus

THE LONG BACKS OF PHARAOHS

The upright posture of the early civilizations is also apparent in Egyptian artifacts. At the entrance of the museum's Egypt exhibit, I admired a giant stone pharaoh while hearing the audio guide's voice explain through the headset, "Around 3000 BC, the wealth and cohesive social system gave rise to the pharaoh dynasties."

I saw inscriptions showcasing the Egyptian people doing manual work like rowing boats, harvesting crops, and carrying heavy bricks—and all depicted a good body posture. These artifacts show long spines, relaxed shoulders, toned abdomens, and pelvic bones aligned under the shoulders. Egyptian hieroglyphics and statues give us an insight into their excellent postural health.

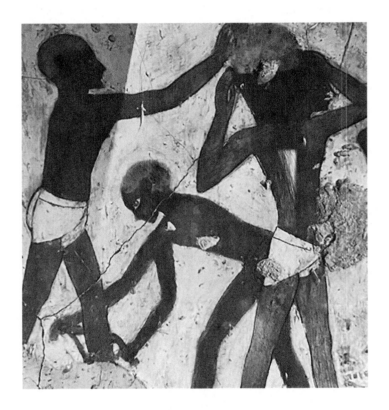

Caption: Posture of Egyptian Workers

"What we see on the artwork in the temples, the walls of tombs, and in paintings on papyrus is that the Egyptian civilization's ideal image of the human body comes pretty close to our western ideals like the modern supermodels of the nineties," says Dr. Franziska Naether joining me for an interview from Germany. Dr. Naether is a professor of Egyptology at the University of Leipzig. According to her, Egyptians strived to have an ideal posture. She specifies, "Looking at the sculptures, we know that they wanted straight backs because it conveys an image of authority and power for the pharaohs, the queens, and of course, the gods." The chair was a symbol of prestige in their culture, and only priests and pharaohs had access to chairs and desks.

ALONG THE RIVER INDUS

Human settlement spread from Africa and West Asia to the northern Persian plateau and eventually entered South Asia. An organized cultural and political entity, the Indus Valley Civilization, flourished around the river Indus in South Asia around 3300 BC. As primarily farming communities, the people of this civilization had a physically laborious job working outside the home. As a result, they emphasized postural health and holistic well-being. An ancient Indus Valley physician named Sushruta incorporated the concepts of physical yogic practice as prescription medicine (Tipton 2008). A compilation of these medical tenets, the *Sushruta Samhita*, outlines, "Exercise is absolutely conducive to a better preservation of health" (Bhishagratna 2018).

The *Sushruta Samhita* frequently expressed concern that a more sedentary lifestyle attained from agricultural advancement would lead to obesity, the root cause of many diseases. It states, "Diseases fly from the presence of a person habituated to regular physical exercise."

Yoga was developed early on as a form of exercise and pre-scribed as a medicine to preserve health and musculoskeletal fitness. The most practiced yogic methods focus on achieving steadiness and strength of the body.

While the Indus Valley Civilization was one of the first civilizations found to have emphasized exercise and its relationship to posture, other civilizations also embraced these concepts.

GREEK GYMNASIUMS

Agriculture and settlement also spread to the continent of Europe. Physical exercise started to become a norm for the Greeks by the time of Homer. In fact, exercise was a civic duty. Gymnasiums established by city-states became com-monplace. In their poems, Homer and other sources describe athletic competitions like boxing, wrestling, discus, spearing, and archery. Athletic training was equated with medicine to fight off illness and promote health. In his treatise *Gymnas-ticus*, Philostratus wrote, "They lifted weights, raced horses and hares, bent or straightened metal bars, pulled plows or carts, lifted bulls and wrestled lions, or swam in the sea to exercise their arms and their entire body" (Nakou 2017).

The results of implementing exercise and having an active life are visible in the impeccable posture depicted in their statues and artwork. The earliest ancient Greeks created limestone sculptures that show human figures with their arms by their sides, long spines, straight legs, squared shoulders, pelvises under their hips, and heads aligned on top of their spines.

Overall, we can see that the importance of body movement via exercise to improve muscle strength, eliminate illnesses, and achieve health was a common belief among earlier civilizations.

INCORPORATE EXERCISE

People in ancient civilizations preserved their posture by making exercise part of their lives. The usual burning question in the mind of many of my clients is, how can I incorporate thirty minutes of exercise into my already busy schedule? If you've already committed to a side business, a writing class, or socializing with friends, you might be surprised to hear you can exercise without giving up any of these activities. Even if you are busy or working from home, there are many ways to add exercise to your daily routine. They are:

Reward Yourself: Exercise while watching TV, YouTube videos, or listening to podcasts. Grab a yoga mat and perform some squats, lunges, and push-ups. You can even follow along with a personal trainer's video on YouTube. There is a plethora of fitness videos out there that can help you get started.

Use the Onsite Gym: Many offices and residential complexes have an onsite fitness center. If you have access to one, try to stack thirty minutes on either end of your day to use the fitness facility and exercise. Using the gym at your workplace is convenient and saves time.

Setup a Desk Station: If you work from home or cannot get away from your desk, you should consider setting up a home office workout station. You can learn more about how to set one up in the insert "setting up your desk station." Keeping the workout equipment handy and visible will motivate you to move, even if it is just in small intervals when you're seated. There are many exercises in the last three chapters of this book you can do without ever leaving your desk.

UPSHOT OF ANCIENT POSTURE

The upshot of exploring ancient lifestyles is that these civilizations exercised and maintained an active lifestyle to preserve their natural posture. Early civilized humans made tools, lived as nomadic hunter-gatherers, and settled around Indus, Nile, and Euphrates riverbanks. The earliest urban settlements placed immense value on public health. The people of these civilizations believed a long spine and proper posture were crucial for power, strength, and better health.

Posture Challenge: I invite you to add some physical exercise to your busy day. Find a type of movement you enjoy. It's high time we follow the wisdom of our ancestors and start incorporating movement to preserve the alignment of our bodies.

CHAPTER 4

1,000 Ways to Sit

———

Childhood memories are some of the most precious keepsakes dear to my heart, and trips to Multan, Pakistan—where my grandmother's family lived—are among my fondest memories. I find much joy in remembering my grandmother's love and the simplicity of being a kid.

"Dadi, the food is delicious," I told my great-grandmother, who was seated in a deep squat on the floor while cooking. My dad, uncles, aunts, and I gathered around on the kitchen floor and ate dinner while seated on chowkis, a type of low Indian stool, to savor the food and each other's company. My grandmother and her family would sit in a deep squat or kneel while resting and doing household chores like dishwashing, cooking, and laundry.

Interestingly, the deep squat is a primary mode of sitting for many people all around the world. When you travel the streets of China or Indonesia, you'll notice people selling food, reading, and waiting, all while crouched in a low squat position. Drop your hips below the knees with your butt nearly touching the ground while keeping the spine extended to get into this worldwide resting position. The deep squat has its roots in the ancient yoga practice. It was once the way we all sat before the invention of the office chair.

DEEP SQUAT: ANOTHER WAY TO SIT

"I don't know why, but my heels don't touch the ground when I go into this deep squatting position," Maureen said in my yoga class.

Leading yoga classes in the park during warm months is usually the highlight of my summers. The natural ambience of the park, with the breeze gliding through the blades of grass and birds singing in the trees, refreshes me. The class participants open their bodies with different rejuvenating asanas. Garland pose or deep squat is a staple in my yoga classes because it has the grounding quality of downward energy flow. It calms our body and brain. But when I direct my class to go into the deep floor squat, many yogis, like Maureen, struggle with the pose.

In much of the developed world, chairs have replaced the deep squat as the primary resting mode. We sit in office chairs, dining chairs, commute in car seats, and watch entertainment from couches. Our bodies have forgotten how to get into a deep squat.

Although poor postural health is a recent concern, research on human posture isn't. Dr. Gordon Hewes, one of the earliest anthropologists to document the postures of cultures all over the globe, was interested in human evolution and cultural postures from an early age. He persisted in his field of study, earning a degree in anthropology at UC Berkley and traveling the globe to study the posture of 480 cultures (Kaschube and Quiatt 1998).

Hewes discovered cultures worldwide had very few postures in common. Instead, people's environments determined the body positions they adopted. Nevertheless, he noted, "At least a fourth of mankind habitually takes a load off its feet by crouching in a deep squat, both at rest and work" (Hewes 1957).

"The human body," he wrote, "can assume something on the order of 1,000 different steady postures." Many cultures assume unique postures that are not practiced in the technological world today. Those postures include variations of the cross-legged position, deep squat, and kneeling. However, industrialized cultures have likely forgone these positions. Instead, they sit all day in chairs, which eventually contributes to a trend of bad postural health in these cultures.

STRENGTH OF SHERPAS

Kenneth Silber's observations of postural differences on his Annapurna Circuit trekking trip through Nepal in 2019 were consistent with that of Gordon Hewes.

Silber, an American journalist and trekker, spoke to me on Zoom. "I had to sign some papers, fill out some forms just for local government; the government officials and I were kneeling or squatting in a field while filling those [papers]," he said, referring to the indigenous communities in Nepal.

Before this strenuous trek, he had signed up for Sherpa support. He had no idea what that meant. He found out when eight indigenous porters came to carry his family's luggage for days of trekking. "A woman, one of the Sherpas, who was quite short with squat ankles and wrists, came and picked up our two hefty bags and walked off with them," Silber said, recalling that day. "I was embarrassed I didn't carry my bag and had this small woman do it." With a grateful smile, he added, "But she did it so effortlessly."

Sherpas, members of a Nepali indigenous tribe, can carry up to 120 percent of their body weight suspended with straps across their foreheads up and down high-altitude mountains, year after year, without injuries (Sohn 2017). These sherpas use their natural posture to protect their spine and other joints while carrying heavy loads.

Environmental adaptation is the only way to explain the Sherpas' high strength. The strength their bodies develop from continually trekking on steep mountain tops keeps their posture unhunched. The discovery of these postural differences further echoes the importance of considering environmental and cultural factors in the understanding of human posture and overall health.

Walk Uphill Like Sherpas: *We can implement the Sherpa posture training by regularly walking or running uphill. Uphill ambulation is one of the best ways to strengthen the posterior muscles of our legs, which are often inactive during deskbound office work. Strong posterior chain muscles improve our body posture and back health.*

SITTING POSTURE OF HUNTER-GATHERERS

Like Sherpas, many African tribespeople enjoy similar postural health. Across Africa, people pursue many activities while squatting on the floor. Dr. David Raichlen, a researcher at the University of Southern California (USC), seeks to understand the evolutionary biology of human resting postures. To achieve this, he and his team studied the Hadza, a group of contemporary Tanzanian hunter-gatherers.

In their study, the Hadza wore devices that tracked physical activity and rest periods. These devices revealed they engaged in high levels of physical activity—over three times the recommended minimum of twenty-two minutes per day by the US health department (Raichlen et al. 2020). However, the Hadza also had high levels of inactivity, comparable to industrialized societies' inactivity levels.

Dr. Raichlen found, "Even though there were long periods of inactivity, one of the key differences we noticed is the Hadza often rest in postures that require their muscles to maintain light activity levels—either in a squat or kneeling." In short, not all sitting positions are equal in terms of their effect on our bodies.

Deep squatting, for example, involves more muscle activity than sitting, leading to consistent activation throughout the day. It leads to full compression and movement of three critical joints: the hips, knees, and ankles. Specialists refer to this as the triple flexion movement, which involves bending at all three joints while folding the tailbone under the body. The key to sitting in a deep squat is the flexibility of muscles around these joints.

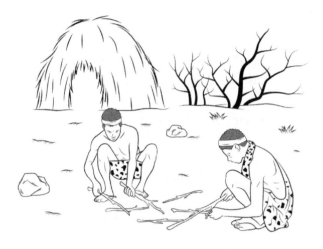

Caption: Hadza Tribe Squatting and Kneeling

Ankle joint flexibility plays a vital role in deep squatting.
People who find it hard to squat with feet flat on the floor
have inflexible ankles. For instance, a toddler's ankle flexibility while dorsiflexing (bending your foot with toes pointing
toward shins) is seventy degrees, while a deskbound professional's flexibility is thirty degrees. As a result, squatting as
a toddler who practices this posture isn't challenging but
is very difficult for a deskbound adult. Dr. Raichlen's team
discovered the ability directly links to a person's metabolic
health, with a low incidence of diabetes and cardiovascular
disease. But is that all we can learn about postural health
from today's indigenous tribes?

There's more. Indigenous tribes also have a 50 to 70 percent
lower rate of back pain (Volinn 1997). In fact, one of the tribes

in central India reports never experiencing it. These people's spinal discs show no sign of degeneration. Comparatively, back pain affects 577 million modern deskbound workers globally (International Association for the Study of Pain 2021).

MODERN-DAY INDIGENOUS POSTURES

Why is there such a vast gap in back pain rates between technological and agricultural cultures?

Biochemist and acupuncturist Dr. Esther Gokhale, from Palo Alto, California, was curious about cultures outside the Western Hemisphere and has studied many indigenous cultures.

In our interview, she told me, "I've studied many village cultures in Burkina Faso, Africa, Brazil, India, Ecuador, Thailand, Portugal, and Southern Europe. You know, you still find some old-world posture in places like Italy, France, and even Portugal, too."

In Africa, she observed women carry heavy water buckets on their heads for long distances and squat while weaving for hours with no back pain. "The first thing that strikes us is that there's something very sound, relaxed, and strong [about their posture]," Dr. Gokhale remarked, specifying that their tall and natural body alignment helps their bodies move effortlessly. "A lot of things are intact in their bodies, natural self-possession, natural dignity, natural beauty. That mixture of being strong and relaxed is very compelling."

She noticed the spinal shape of these tribal people was different from western populations. Instead, their spines are much flatter and more elongated. With these observations in mind, she started practicing walking, sitting, and standing in a J-shaped spine to help her back pain. Her back pain disappeared. This experience inspired her to develop the Gokhale Method. Today, many Gokhale Method-certified bodywork practitioners are helping their clients live pain-free.

"Most of these communities might not have the intellectual knowledge, but they have kinesthetic knowledge of how to be in their bodies," she said.

You can see in the picture below that the indigenous farmer is doing a more physically demanding task but has a better posture than the less physically active person sitting in front of a laptop. The sitting woman's posture is more fatiguing than the female farmer's posture.

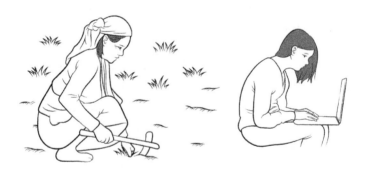

Caption: Indigenous Farmer's Posture Versus Deskbound Posture

Dr. Hewes, Mr. Silber, Dr. Raichlen, and Dr. Gokhale all observed the benefits of assuming common ancient postures. In many societies, even today, postural health is emphasized intuitively. They have discovered that adopting different sitting and standing postures is a way to keep our muscles working in harmony to fight the forces of gravity and maintain an unhunched posture.

ADOPTING THE INDIGENOUS WAY TO SIT

Sitting in one position, like in an office chair, is one of the most critical postural problems facing us today. It creates a perfect storm of muscle tension. The Hadza tribe example is evidence that chair sitting decreases muscle activity. Dr. Gokhale's research shows us our postural habits lead to tight muscles in our back and lower back pain.

Thankfully, there is an easy way to increase muscle flexibility and activity: vary your sitting positions often. Change your sitting position every thirty to forty minutes from regular chair sitting to a cross-legged position and from sitting on the chair to sitting on the floor. This will do wonders for your body.

You can instantly set up a floor desk station on a carpet or rug in your office. Pick any floor desk higher than sixteen inches and about thirty-six inches in length. I use my standing desk attachment, which works as a floor desk as well. At first, you might feel stiff because a healthy posture might feel foreign to your muscles. Try using a thin cushion for padding and comfort. Sitting on the floor improves posture and awareness. You can learn more about how to setup a floor desk station and find my floor desk suggestions at www.aeshatahir.com/books. You can also find them in the resource section at the end of this book.

While on the floor, tune into your inner yogi. Try different sitting positions like a deep squat, kneeling, and butterfly position (heels touching and pulling in with knees out to sides). If you're not comfortable getting into these positions, worry not. You only need to hold these sitting positions for short intervals to enjoy their benefits. Even ten to fifteen minutes of sitting in these positions will help get your body limber. With consistent practice, your muscles become more flexible, allowing you to stay seated for more extended periods.

The benefits of practicing a variety of sitting positions are manifold.

- It increases the number of muscles recruited during the work, balancing the workload distribution on different body parts.

- It lifts the weight off your lower back and lengthens the spine.

- It increases oxygenated blood to muscles, which reduces tiredness usually experienced by deskbound workers.

Practicing sitting positions on the floor is the secret behind indigenous cultures' long, functional, healthy lives.

POSTURE FOR LONGEVITY

"I'm getting old," many clients tell me while going through the functional activity test. During the test, my clients attempted to pick up their shoes from the floor and put them on while standing and without support, but most of them couldn't do it. These clients are healthy adults who can engage in activities like dancing, running, walking, and biking. They, however, struggle with this simple test due to demineralization and muscle weakness.

As you learned earlier in this chapter, people of indigenous tribes seldom experience poor mobility due to age. I personally witnessed my great-grandmother squat on the floor without any help until she was ninety-eight years young.

So, can poor posture impact our life expectancy? That was the question on the mind of a group of scientists led by Dr. Deborah Kado, MD, at the UCLA school of medicine. Her team discovered a hunched-back posture more than doubles the risk of death from respiratory and cardiovascular diseases (Kado et al. 2004). Thus, the restricted body position of a deskbound worker leads to immobility and conditions that can shorten our lifespan.

SITTING AND RISING TEST FOR MORTALITY

Your posture can predict your mortality. A Brazilian physician, Dr. Claudio Gil Araujo, and his colleagues have developed a Sitting-Rising Test to help predict mortality.

This test is valid for all age groups, and all it requires is to go from a standing position to a cross-legged seated position on the ground. If you have orthopedic issues, it is important to perform this test with a movement specialist.

To perform this test:

- Start in a standing position

- Your starting score is ten points

- Cross your feet and lower into a seated position on the floor without touching your body, the floor, or any walls

- Any time you touch an object, you lose a point

- If you lose your balance or wobble at any time, you lose half a point

- Try to stand back up the same way you sat down

- The process of scoring as you stand up is the same as getting down

- A score of ten is a sign of seamless mobility. The lower the score, the higher the risk of death

- Each point decreases your all-cause mortality rate by 21 percent (De Brito et al. 2012)

- A score of three or less increases your risk of death by fivefold (De Brito et al. 2012)

- The video for this test is accessible at www.aeshatahir.com/books

Our functional ability to sit and stand off the floor is directly related to the flexibility of our muscles. The more flexible our muscles, the easier it is to keep our natural posture, and finding your natural posture can help you live a longer and more functional life.

UPSHOT OF SITTING ON THE FLOOR

In our society, we might think the only way to work is by sitting in chairs. However, the history of indigenous populations and their practices in modern times reveals many other ways to sit or rest that can benefit our bodies. In our modern work-driven culture, we blame reduced flexibility on old age. But old age isn't the biggest contributor to our postural issues. The real culprits are unhealthy resting behaviors and environments. Unfortunately, comfortable deep squatting is a forgotten posture in technological societies. Different ways to sit—including kneeling, cross-legged, and a deep passive squat—are not just good for us but are embedded in our physiology. Longevity, then, is a result of respecting our physiology.

CHAPTER 5

It Starts Young

"There was no possibility of playing today," said my disappointed son while hopping into the car.

When they tell you there is no possibility, they are wrong. As adults, it is our collective responsibility to create opportunities for children to be healthy and grow into healthy adults.

The camp counselor, seeing the puzzled look on my face, followed with, "I want to let you know we give technology breaks to kids at the camp. Your kids are welcome to bring their phones and iPads to the camp. I noticed they didn't have those with them today."

I shared my thoughts with the camp counselor and suggested the camp provide an option for kids to play in the gym in addition to the various activities available to them. My kids enjoy summer camps. They make many new friends and spend each day doing different activities. But using mobile devices at camp was a first.

Was sending my children to summer camp without phones only about technology? No. It was about the poor posture kids develop from a very young age.

MODERN CHILDREN'S PHYSICAL HEALTH

Sitting with poor postures while using phones and other mobile devices strains children's backs, necks, and shoulders, affecting their overall physical health. Nearly one million elementary and middle school children in California are too physically weak and out of breath to pass a basic fitness test that includes running, lifting, and stretching (Asimov 2012). The committee for the United States Report Card on Physical Activity for Children and Youth measures children's health based on these indicators:

- Overall physical activity

- Sedentary behaviors

- Active transportation

- Organized sport participation

- Active play

- Health-related fitness

- Family and peers

In 2018, this report card issued a "D-" grade for the health of youth nationwide (National Physical Activity Plan 2018).

It's easy to see we are passing a technology-heavy lifestyle on to our children, predisposing them to poor posture and associated health risks as they grow. Failing the fitness test indicates inadequate muscle strength, poor posture control, and balance. Three decades after the worldwide web's launch and our children can barely meet the physical activity guidelines set by the US Department of Health. For our kids, it's not just the biological effects of poor posture.

Increased hunched sitting time is directly related to inferior grades in high school students. Students who score higher grades regularly engage in physical activity for an average of sixty minutes daily (CDC Healthy Schools 2021).

How much time are our children spending in a hunched-over seated position? According to a Commonsense Media research study funded by the US government, children ages eight and under spend 3.5 hours daily sitting and consuming media on different digital devices (Common Sense Media 2011). By age eighteen, this time increases to 7.5 hours daily (Tsukayama 2015). Seven and a half hours on top of the time they spend sitting at school. Before the technological age, kids would go out to play soccer and hockey with their friends. Now they go to basements to play with friends online. If they are involved in sports, they text and watch social media while in a slumped posture on the sidelines.

Children today aren't receiving the physical stimulus necessary to naturally develop their muscles and joints for a healthy upright posture. And as we've learned, good posture is essential for the well-being of the entire body.

THE MOVEMENT CONNECTION

As I stand outside the elementary school building on a nice spring afternoon, young runners surround me. They run the half-mile loop around the school's perimeter, talking to their friends happily. Their red cheeks and broad smiles prove how much fun they're having. I can feel their endorphins coursing through the air.

Since 2019, I have been organizing the annual eight-week after-school running program at my children's elementary school. A nonprofit organization, iRun4Life, supports this program. As a runner, I find it fulfilling to share my passion for running with children. There is no better feeling than watching a child who could barely walk a half-mile loop finish a 3K race with a medal after just eight weeks of practice. As a running coach, I have the privilege of seeing these transformations frequently.

As I coach the runners during their practice, I notice their gait, which is how a person walks and runs. Over the years, I have observed many older kids show deteriorated movement patterns in fifth and sixth grade. Most of them hit the ground hard with their heels, and their foot comes down with force. I see many children running with their feet turned out and knees turned in. Some have shrimp back posture while running. These postural distortions can increase the risk of injury, which is concerning because running is a part of most of the land sports our kids play. Plus, the way our kids run and walk impacts their other activities as well. Even if these changes aren't visible right away, the consequences of poor movement patterns are visible years later in young adults.

Dr. James Carter, a chiropractic doctor and the former governor of the Australian Spinal Research Foundation, warns us that children who hunch over phones for extended periods can develop spinal deformities in the neck region. He often sees many young patients with poor posture who fail a simple heel-to-toe test and tend to fall over. The heel-to-toe test is a standard test used to check a person's balance. In this test, the patient walks along a straight line with the toes of the back foot touching the heel of the front foot at each step. An unsteady gait while performing the test is an indicator of poor posture.

He is not the only one to warn us of the effect of poor posture on children's health. Dr. Rupa Chakravarty, physical therapy doctor at Root Cause Medical writes in an article, "I am alarmed at the rapidly increasing number of children with poor posture. In addition to poor posture, the number of children coming in to see me for spinal problems and muscle problems that had typically only been prevalent in adults has risen markedly" (Chakravarty 2021). In fact, between 25–60 percent of children and adolescents show posture distortions like rounded shoulders, tilted heads, and low back arches (David et al. 2021).

Over the past few decades, our kids have become competent at slouching while sitting and moving. Access to technology has accelerated our unfortunate progress in this field. However, we can help our kids learn how to walk and run properly and encourage them to get involved in physical activity to help prevent postural distortions and improve overall health as they grow.

WALK IT OUT

We can do this by helping kids develop proper gait patterns through walking, translating to improved performance in running and other sports. Walking involves every part of the body, from the feet to the head, so it's important to focus on each aspect.

Heel to Toe: Each step should begin with the heel, rolling through the arch and to the toes. Encourage kids to avoid striking the heel too far back and hard. Instead, the heel should connect to the ground softly and roll the foot forward. The final push-off should be with their toes.

Engage the Core: Squeezing the back leg muscles, glutes, and hamstrings during forward movement will keep their core muscles engaged.

Lengthen the Back: Direct them to keep their backs long by avoiding a forward lean and rounding of their shoulders.

Balance the Head: Looking at the horizon is the best way to correct children's moving posture. I tell children to imagine they are puppets and a string hanging from the sky is pulling their heads. They immediately balance their head over the spine, and their chin runs parallel to the floor.

Swing the Arms: A back-and-forth swing of arms by their midsection is the best way to get the whole body in motion.

By teaching the kids proper walking techniques, we can help them adopt a healthy posture and decrease the risk of injury while playing sports and later on in life. Many of my clients ask me if their musculoskeletal alignment issues are inherited. I ask them to bring their childhood picture as a young toddler at the next visit. When they bring the picture, we can all see their posture relaxed and flawless.

POSTURE LESSONS FROM A TODDLER

Next time you see a toddler, notice their perfectly relaxed posture: ears behind the collar bones, shoulders back, a natural arch in the back, and a long supple spine. They naturally sit into a deep squat.

"Now you may have noticed when young children pick things up from the ground, they drop down into this perfect squat," says Roger Frampton, author of *The Flexible Body*, from the TED stage in 2016.

Their effortless posture while sitting and standing isn't the only beautiful thing. The way they move with perfectly stacked spines is also noteworthy. They hinge at their hips while supporting their backs to reach for their toys.

Toddlers have an intuitively unstrained posture. The fact that they carry their weight over their hips and joints so optimally proves it's our body's primal posture. As babies and toddlers, we have a naturally pain-free posture, and our bodies can form a fluid stance with play.

Frampton describes a toddler depicted on the screen near him, saying, "Unfortunately, as a consequence of our current human conditioning, this natural resting position is about to be taken away from this child. He's about to be taught that a resting position is a chair." Once our children are school-age, they become exposed to lengthy chair-sitting episodes.

DESKBOUND IN SCHOOLS

Schools have many benefits for kids. As an advocate of structured education and the school system, I believe my children benefit from different forms of education the school provides, like social and emotional skills, knowledge, and leadership skills. Unfortunately, sitting in chairs for hours isn't one of those benefits.

At the turn of the twentieth century, some parents became increasingly concerned about their school-aged children's posture (Joyce 2014). They didn't want their kids to attend school because they were worried about the kids sitting behind their desks for six hours at a stretch. At the time, school attendance was becoming mandatory. These laws met much resistance, and every component of attending school came under scrutiny.

Doctors campaigned on the premise that modern furniture, such as cramped school desks, will lead to physical deformations. As a result, posture training became part of school education.

In the early twentieth century, the American Posture League was formed to promote posture education. Jessie Bancroft, a president of the league, wrote in her book *The Posture of School Children* that "Erect carriage of the body is necessary for full vigor and health, to prevent waste of energy in maintaining the upright position in any of the activities of life, with children, to admit of proper growth and development" (Yosifon and Stearns 1998).

Schools eventually began using evaluation techniques and corrective exercises to straighten kids' spines and correct postural irregularities. Students with perfect upright postures received posture pins. This posture movement peaked in the 1940s when the military performed posture evaluations to see if potential soldiers were fit to join the armed forces. They saw good posture as a sign of good health.

A century ago, the United States was a frontrunner in posture education. Kids received lessons about ergonomics, body mechanics, and posture correction exercises in grade school. However, these programs were short-lived.

POP POSTURE: THE NEW NORM

In the late 1960s, the posture movement started fading out. Conflicting cultural values and norms were one of the primary reasons that posture education in schools started to decline. The methods used to evaluate and reinforce the posture in schools came under scrutiny. Parents didn't want the revealing photos of their children in school records to document posture progress. Also, protecting the privacy of images was becoming more complex with technological advances.

Finally, the growing counterculture movement normalized hunching over as the "cool" resting posture. People began to slouch while gathering around the radio, and slumping into the couches became the style. They saw straight body posture as rigid and authoritative. Eventually, school systems phased out posture programs at schools.

Today, there is a crucial need for the revival of these programs in our schools—especially considering that research shows higher effectiveness of posture correction programs when children are young and still growing (Candotti et al. 2013).

SCHOOL ERGONOMICS

A Kinnarps survey conducted in Swedish schools found 40 percent of pupils don't feel comfortable sitting on their chairs (Kinnarps n.d.). This discomfort can morph into poor posture habits and potential health issues in the long run. We know classrooms are one of the most important environments for children's learning and development, so we should ensure they are designed for better posture to improve children's health.

Fortunately, there are many tools out there in the market that can create posture-positive classrooms. For instance, stands for laptops and mobile devices that can bring the screens up to students' eye levels are one such tool that can significantly improve children's posture. Portable desk converters that rise to a standing desk's height and are easily adjustable to eye-level are another cost-effective classroom tool. Allowing children to stand at their desks keeps their muscles and joints relaxed and flexible. I share more details on these resources in the resource section of this book.

BETTER POSTURE STARTS AT HOME

Better posture education for kids can start at home, especially considering poor posture is often a result of lifelong habits. As parents and caregivers, we can introduce our kids to healthy posture and help them build positive habits they can carry into adulthood. A few tips for developing these habits follow below.

Educate Kids: Teaching children about good posture while sitting and standing is the first step in helping them adopt proper posture. Using visual aids like picture books and cartoon characters helps children get the concept. *Posture Posey and the Slumpyback Goblins* is a good children's posture book.

Ergonomic Workstation at Home: Make sure your child has a workspace that encourages good posture. Using props to customize the furniture for your child's comfort can prevent slouching over homework. For example, use a chair with firm seating, place a rolled blanket or cushion to bring the backrest closer to the child's back, use a hamper or storage box as the footrest, and use firm pillows to raise the seat's height. While setting up an ergonomically sound workstation for children, ensure that:

- Their elbows, hips, and knees are bent at ninety degrees

- Their backs are straight and resting comfortably against the back of a chair

- Their feet are planted in front of them on a firm surface

- The screen is at eye level to avoid bending their necks to look down

Schedule Movement Breaks: Children naturally have the urge to move often and have shorter attention spans. Schedule movement breaks of five to ten minutes in their routine every twenty minutes. Building lots of movement into the daily routine gives children the physiologic and mental health benefits of increased blood circulation and oxygen levels.

Encourage Varying Positions: Children like to assume many different positions that adults avoid, like kneeling, squatting, and lying down on their stomachs. Encourage kids to work in these positions while ensuring that their necks and backs are supported. Encourage your kids to read, write, and watch TV while standing. Remember to raise the screen to eye level in a standing position.

Developing these small habits can go a long way.

UPSHOT OF YOUNG POSTURE

Children are born with natural postures before being introduced to restrictive sitting and adapting accordingly. Unfortunately, that means adapting to poor posture habits. Implementing a posture education program at school can improve the health of future generations. Parents and caregivers can play their part by introducing positive posture habits to kids at home.

Posture Challenge: To start teaching better posture habits, make one of the changes suggested in this chapter each week.

You can lead by example and demonstrate good posture for others to see. Keep a long back with properly aligned shoulders and hips. Remember, young children are constantly observing and emulating us.

Acquiring positive postural habits during their developmental years will help our kids stay with the practice for the rest of their lives.

The BRACE Posture Correction Model

Parts two and three of the book explain the BRACE model for posture correction. BRACE stands for breath, relaxation, activity, and corrective exercise. The way we breathe, manage stress, and move can impact our posture and health. Incorporating these aspects as part of posture correction model reinforces proper body mechanics that put less stress on our body as we move.

BRACE

POSTURE CORRECTION FRAMEWORK

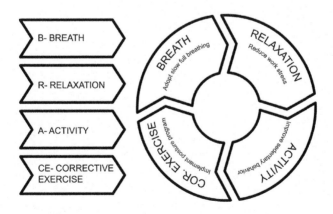

- B- BREATH
- R- RELAXATION
- A- ACTIVITY
- CE- CORRECTIVE EXERCISE

BREATH — Adopt slow full breathing

RELAXATION — Reduce work stress

ACTIVITY — Improve sedentary behavior

COR. EXERCISE — Implement posture program

PART 2

BREATH, RELAXATION, ACTIVITY

CHAPTER 6

Breathing Shapes
Our Body

———

"Just relax" was the mantra repeating in her head as she slowly pushed herself into the depths of the sea (Murphy 2020). Trying to ignore the pressure rising in her ears and abdomen, she frantically kicked her feet. Sunrays trickled down through the ocean water, and she could see the shipwreck below—her target. But all she could think about was breathing.

Jen Murphy is a free diver in Maui, Hawaii. She loves to explore treasures under the sea by diving into its depths. But to access this kind of treasure, plunging a hundred feet below sea level is required. Equalizing the pressure under deep water is not an easy task, especially with our built-in habit of shallow breathing. For Jen, learning slow diaphragmatic breathing and activating her lesser-used core muscles are a must to be able to embrace these depths.

Since that dive, breathwork classes at wellness retreats in Maui have been part of her training routine.

Diaphragmatic breathing positively affects our physiology, helping deep divers like Jen. It can change the way we stack our skeleton, facilitating an open and natural posture.

GATEWAY TO LIFE

Breath is life. We can go weeks without food and days without water, but only moments without breath. Yet we don't give much thought to it, even though we take an average of 20,000 breaths daily (Miller 2022).

Like Jen, I'm familiar with the postural effects of breathwork. Because of working at a desk, I often suffered from extreme shortness of breath during running sessions, and the tracker on my watch would show a high breathing rate throughout the day. I decided to sign up for breathwork classes to improve my breathing. The first class I attended was at the Frequency studio in Chelsea, New York. It was an unforgettable experience and changed the way I breathe.

"Let this breath open your mind, body, and soul," the instructor said gently. Her words landed softly like rose petals on the grass over the new world music in the background— breath syncing with the music coming through the headset. I opened my eyes to the virtual constellation above me. My whole body was participating in the breathing process.

I was lying side by side with fifteen other people in a gray dome-shaped chamber, strengthening my lungs. This breathing practice was a massage for my stressed muscles, tendons, and joints. I could feel my spine lengthening and muscles relaxing.

Hooked up on technology today, we ignore breathing, letting it run in the backdrop just like the computer applications we work on. And we are completely unaware of the impact breathing has on our upright posture.

VITALITY OF BREATH

When focusing our attention on the movement of our inhales and exhales, we have a better awareness of our bodies. Our muscles relax as they receive oxygenated nourishment. Relaxed muscles are a prerequisite for better posture.

"I worked as a respiratory physical therapist in the ICUs and Orthopedic wards. I saw how people's breathing was very dysfunctional," Dr. Campbell Will says during our Zoom interview. He founded Breath Body Therapy, a breathwork school for coaches. Through his experience as a therapist and breathwork practitioner, he has learned breath holds the power to better posture. He tells me, "Around that time when I was working in the hospital, I encountered the Wim Hof Method. That was my first introduction to the wealth of conscious breathwork." Wim Hof is a breathwork teacher and an extreme athlete. His breathing method promotes relaxation, body temperature control, increased immunity, reduced stress, and increased focus.

"In my practice, I have seen time and again that breathing practices can empower individuals with the understanding of postural tension, which is tied in with self-regulation of stress symptoms," Dr. Will shares further with a smile. "Through the lens of the objective understanding of what's going on in the body when we breathe quickly or slowly or deep or shallow, we can understand the impact breath has on our health."

AWARENESS OF BREATH

Investigating breathing mechanics is important to understand how your breath impacts posture. Here is an exercise that can help you differentiate between chest and diaphragmatic breathing:

Lie down with your back on the floor, with knees bent and hips soft, and rest one hand on your chest and one hand on your belly. Breathe in and out the way you regularly do a few times. Which hand feels the movement? Take note of that hand.

If the hand on your belly rises more than the hand on your chest, then kudos on using your core muscles for breathing. But, if your hand on the chest rises more than the one on your belly, you take short, shallow breaths most of the time. When you take shallow breaths, you use your upper body muscles like shoulders and chest. The overactivity of these muscles is related to our distorted deskbound posture.

BREATHING MECHANICS

Many muscles are involved in this process, like the breathing action of expanding and contracting the belly and the chest. The muscles attached to the ribcage are also part of the respiratory process. Our inspiratory muscles expand the rib cage and help bring air to our lungs. Our expiratory muscles compress the thoracic cavity and let the air out of our lungs. Below is more information about the many muscles that aid in breathing:

- Lungs are the primary respiratory muscle with an elastic capacity (Calais-Germain 2006).

- The diaphragm is a dome-shaped muscle just beneath the lungs that separates the chest and abdominal cavities.

- The external and internal intercostals are the slender muscles between our ribs.

- The pectoralis minor is the small chest muscle that lies next to the ribcage and helps elevate the ribs.

- The abdominal muscles attach to the ribcage and stabilize the entire abdominal region during exhalation.

- Sternocleidomastoid and scalene muscles are the secondary breathing muscles in our neck and help elevate the clavicle bones and rib cage during inhalation.

I wanted to learn more about how our muscle activity while breathing figured into the relationship with upright posture. To find those answers, I headed to Jefferson Hospital in Philadelphia on a sunny Friday afternoon. As I passed the glass building of the Emergency Room, I saw paramedics pushing their patients. My thoughts drifted to the COVID-19 pandemic and so many patients who suffered a respiratory collapse due to the virus.

Seated on a green bench in the hospital's garden, surrounded by the pansy flowers in front of Sidney Kimmel Cancer Center's glass walls, I offered gratitude for my respiratory health. The vitality of my breath became even more apparent to me in those few minutes. As I took a slow breath and looked up, I saw Dr. Jeffrey Hoag, the Section Chief of Pulmonary Medicine, walking toward me.

When I asked him about breathing, he said, "The diaphragm is the big muscle that helps us breathe when it contracts. It happens unconsciously most of the time." When we breathe in, he explained, the diaphragm and the intercostal muscles of the ribs contract, expanding the lungs. The ribs push out as they lift away from the hips. This expansion increases air volume inside the lungs with a decrease in air pressure inside the lungs. The decreased air pressure in the lungs causes the air to flow into the lungs and completes the inhalation process.

Inhalation is closely related to the position of our spine, which dictates our posture. Our ribs are attached to different spinal discs. Optimal inward breathing elongates the spine, reducing pressure on the intervertebral discs and strengthening our core muscles.

"[Our] breathing mechanism is designed to work best if we're upright and in a standing position," says Dr. Hoag. Standing is better than sitting down because it allows the abdomen to expand. The relaxation of the diaphragm and intercostal muscles follows this action. While standing, the diaphragm relaxes like an elastic balloon with the help of gravity. The diaphragm pulls the chest down to create a negative intrathoracic pressure, bringing air through our mouth and nose.

DYSFUNCTIONAL BREATHING AND DESKBOUND PEOPLE
Talking about breathing in a seated position, he says, "When we're sitting down, the abdominal pressure is higher because

our legs are flexed, and they are pushing up our abdomen, and so the diaphragm has to work harder to expand the thorax. So when that happens, we recruit the accessory respiratory muscles of the chest wall and the neck muscles for respiration." These muscles compensate as lung expanders.

Imagine blowing a balloon into a narrow coke bottle versus a gallon milk jug. The balloon's ability to inflate is relative to the space around it. Similarly, our lungs can't expand with a compressed abdomen in an office chair.

When the chest, shoulder, and neck muscles are called upon to do the work of the diaphragm, these muscles get overworked and tight. These tight, overworked muscles result in rounded shoulders and a hunched-over posture for deskbound professionals.

Better Breathing Hack: Use a standing desk for half of your working hours. Standing allows us to engage our lungs and expand ribs to the front, sides, and back. This movement of ribs lengthens the muscles along the spine, orienting our body along the line of gravity.

OPEN POSTURE THROUGH BETTER BREATHING

Proper breathing is the first step toward easing the tension in our upper body and finding our natural and relaxed posture.

Diaphragmatic breathing elongates the spine, increases the space between the joints, and reinforces the spine's natural curves. It reduces the tension in our upper body. In addition to the static posture, diaphragmatic breathing improves our functional posture and increases the spine's ability to twist and bend.

"We'll be working on your breathing for the next eight weeks," I said to Julia. Julia is a financial analyst at a major financial investment bank in New York City. Her work involves commuting to different client sites and sitting in long meetings. She prefers to take a taxi to stack multiple clients during the day. Lately, she has experienced episodic asthma attacks. She went to see an allergy specialist to rule out seasonal allergies. Her allergist created a treatment plan for her asthma and suggested she should improve her posture.

Taking in enough oxygen seems like a simple task, but for people with asthma, it can be a struggle. Approximately twenty-five million Americans have asthma, with more than 3,500 asthma-related deaths each year (Goff 2022).

Julia's rounded shoulder posture promoted overbreathing using her compensatory chest wall muscles. Her continuous overbreathing was the cause of lower levels of carbon dioxide in her body. She is expelling more of it out with every exhale, resulting in inflammation of the airways and muscle spasms and leading to asthma attacks (Campbell, Hoffmann, and Glasziou 2018).

The bent head-neck-chest position of office workers like Julia reduces diaphragm muscle strength, limiting lung capacity by as much as 30 percent (Kang, Jeong, and Choi 2018). The diaphragm can move up to ten centimeters during active cardiorespiratory exercise, but for Julia, it doesn't expand fully (John Hopkins School of Medicine 1995). Offering breathing education to activate the diaphragm and retraining core muscles is my approach to relieving asthma symptoms due to poor posture (Zeltner 2010).

Over the next three months, Julia followed the remedial exercise plan to correct her rounded shoulder posture. She incorporated positive breathing habits during the workday to ease the tightness in her chest muscles. The frequency of her asthma attacks became considerably reduced. When I checked in with her six months after completing her posture correction program, she told me she hadn't experienced an asthma attack in eight weeks.

Posture is essential to healthy breathing and can help relieve breathing conditions like asthma when performed in conjunction with proper medical care.

JUST BREATHE

Breathing to restore healthy posture involves relaxation of our bodies and using the three-dimensional muscles of our respiratory system. Practicing slow breathing is easy and can be done right at your desk. The steps to activate our diaphragm and practice slow breaths are as follows.

- Stand behind your desk or lie down on the floor with your back flat on the ground to expand your abdomen.

- If standing, stack your shoulders over your hips.

- If lying flat on the floor, press your lower back and soles of the feet into the floor.

- Inhale slowly through the nose keeping your shoulders relaxed while lifting your abdomen. Notice that your belly and ribs push forward as you breathe.

- Exhale slowly through your mouth, relaxing your jaw. Continue exhaling until your belly touches your spine.

- Repeat the exercise as many times as you are comfortable.

Diaphragmatic breathing can be practiced twice a day at a minimum or as often as you like. You can access a short video demonstrating diaphragmatic breathing at www.aeshatahir. com/books.

UPSHOT OF DIAPHRAGMATIC BREATHING

Diaphragmatic breathing can relax our muscles and lengthen our spine. As deskbound professionals, shallow breaths weaken our lung muscles over time and lead to upper body tension, worsening slouched posture by rounding the shoulders.

Posture Challenge: If you spend hours behind your computer screen, try incorporating standing work intervals and practicing diaphragmatic breathing. Daily diaphragmatic breathing exercises can reverse the effects of shallow breathing on your body.

CHAPTER 7

Breathing Shapes Our Brain

———

He heard the explosion. All he could see was smoke around him. When he looked down, he was bleeding uncontrollably. His legs had been nearly severed at the knees.

US Marine Corps Officer Jake D. didn't panic when his vehicle drove over an explosive device in Afghanistan. He stayed calm, checked on his men, put tourniquets on his legs, and asked for help before blacking out. Doctors at the hospital told him he would have bled to death if he hadn't stayed calm enough to make those choices. In the moment, Jake remembered the breathing technique he had learned during his training boot camp. That controlled breathing exercise saved his life. Such is the power of breath.

Our breath shapes our brain, which controls how we react and respond in stressful work situations.

OH! THE WORK STRESS

Though the stressors are obviously different, office workers exist in their own kind of combat zone. Bombs may not be raining down, but the never-ending flood of emails can feel that way. Getting put on a new project when you're already working on others might feel like an invasion. The constant demand to juggle deadlines, absent coworkers, and the minutia of the everyday career leaves no room for deskbound professionals to drop their guard and truly relax. The expectation of unceasing efficiency is nearly impossible to meet without sacrificing your health.

All of that stress leaves a physical weight on our bodies. We slump beneath it, never fully relaxing because we are continually under pressure. Chronic stress locks our bodies into rigid postures that activate a sympathetic nervous system response in our brains.

Imagine you are running to catch the bus. Your body needs more oxygen to match your increased activity, so it signals the brain to prompt faster and deeper breathing. This increases the amount of oxygen in the blood. Paired with the oxygen rise is the rise of carbon dioxide (CO_2) levels. To compensate for the accelerated rate of exhalation, your body will increase CO_2 so that it doesn't drop to dangerously low levels. Overall, this process levels the oxygen and CO_2 gases in your blood according to your physical demands.

The same overbreathing response kicks in when you are, say, racing to the next managerial meeting. The small amount of exertion of working on the computer combined with the urgency you experience due to work deadlines also results in faster breathing. When you start taking quick breaths, you're using the muscles in the chest cavity instead of the diaphragm (Services 2015). This leads to low CO_2 levels, making your blood alkaline. This is called *respiratory alkalosis* and contributes to mental fatigue, anxiety, and lower back pain.

In her book, *The New Rules of Posture*, structural integration practitioner Mary Bond puts it this way: "Overbreathing is to air what overeating is to food." Breathing rapidly is as harmful to our bodies as breathing too slowly. She writes, "When someone is breathing rapidly under stress, it's easy to recognize acute hyperventilation [overbreathing], but chronic overbreathing [what office workers experience] often goes undetected."

Over Breathing Cycle

Over breathing leads to tense muscles and poor posture

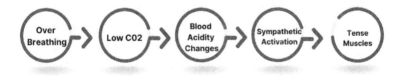

Caption: Overbreathing Cycle in Deskbound Professionals

One of my clients experienced the adverse effects of chronic overbreathing.

"Ms. Conrad, I am here to take your vitals," the ICU nurse said, interrupting Susan's thoughts. It was May 25th, 2021. Susan was on a ventilator, unable to breathe on her own, and experiencing severe air deprivation. Only three days prior, Susan was sitting in the board room of her investment banking firm, attending an executive meeting. Yesterday she was admitted to the hospital with shortness of breath and disabling chest pain. At the hospital, based on her chest radiographs, doctors diagnosed her with severe pneumonia.

She was an otherwise healthy adult with no history of respiratory illnesses. Despite that, her breathing rate was too high, and her pulse oximeter showed a low oxygen concentration.

Two months before this crisis, her investment firm announced they were restructuring the organization. They had started laying off many top-level executives. She was afraid she might be next. She hadn't imagined she would be in the hospital fighting for her life. Susan was a client of mine when she started as a junior investor at the firm, and I have since watched her climb the corporate ladder. It took three weeks of hospitalization before she got better. Susan's story is astonishing, but it is a reminder that overbreathing induced by constant stress can have dire health consequences.

CO2 Hunger: It's a common belief that we only need oxygen to live, and carbon dioxide is just a byproduct. The truth is that carbon dioxide is as important as oxygen, if not more. We inhale to regulate the amount of carbon dioxide in our bodies. Fast breathing eliminates this gas very quickly, leading to air hunger. Our bodies compensate by breathing even faster to achieve optimal levels of carbon dioxide in our bodies. Without the correct levels of CO2, our body will become oxygen deficient.

THE BRAIN'S EMERGENCY ROOM

Our bodies are marvelous machines built to stay in balance in all possible ways. The body's central nervous system is armed with the job of keeping this equilibrium. This system has two main branches: the sympathetic branch, which is our brain's emergency response system designated to keep us safe, and the parasympathetic branch, which is our brain's calming and regeneration center. I like to call it our brain's Zen room.

Work stress can cause the sympathetic nervous system to activate fast breathing. Fast breathing can only be interrupted by activating the Zen room in the parasympathetic nervous system. The vagus nerve connects the brain's calming center to the body. Some of the vagus nerve endings run under our diaphragm muscle. Relaxed, slow, and full breathing stimulates this nerve, which activates the parasympathetic nervous system. In this way, breathing is an optimal tool to break the work stress cycle and allow our minds and muscles to relax. Relaxed muscles are aligned muscles. Breathing slowly molds our body into its natural posture.

BREATHING, THE BRAIN, AND PRODUCTIVITY

I'd be remiss if I talked about work stress, breathing, and the brain but didn't bring up productivity—one of the major concerns for my corporate clients. Organizations always want to improve their bottom lines by increasing employee output.

Office workers also desire to be more efficient in completing their tasks so they have more time for themselves.

When we practice slow breathing, the oxygen supply to our brain increases. This oxygenation of the brain leads to better focus and clarity. Thus, learning how to breathe slowly by engaging our parasympathetic system is vital to increasing productivity for deskbound teams and professionals.

Slowing down and being intentional with breathing improves our concentration by activating our cerebral cortex. Niraj Naik, founder of international breathwork school SOMA Breath and trainer to many breathwork practitioners, says, "The cerebral cortex is the largest region of the cerebrum [the most anterior part of the brain] in the mammalian brain, and plays a key role in memory, attention, perception, cognition, awareness, thought, language, and consciousness (Wheeler 2020)."

Optimal breathing allows proper alignment of our body, making us more resilient to work stress and increasing our efficiency during strenuous tasks. Better focus, resilience to stress, and clarity correlate with higher productivity. Slow breathing also increases productivity by elevating our energy levels. Breath is a channel for energy.

BREATH AND ENERGY

Controlled breathing has its roots in ancient cultures. Many different religious and cultural practices teach breathing techniques, sometimes in the form of prayer and sometimes in the form of meditation.

Ancient Yoga scriptures point to *prana*, Sanskrit for "primary energy." *Pranayama* is the control of energy. Yoga teaches us breathing acts as a bridge, facilitating the connection between body and mind. Kundalini yoga and breathwork expert Eva Kornet said during our zoom interview, "Mentally, emotionally, spiritually, breathwork has an impact on all levels."

Slouched, closed posture is an embodiment of your emotional state. "When you have trauma, you compress your body physically, then you don't exhale," Eva explained. "When you let your body breathe slowly, you release the trauma out of the nervous system. So now you can have a new life experience, and your nervous system becomes more neutral." When you don't exhale fully, you can't release the negative energy, which gets trapped. That's why breathing exercises provide mental clarity and even a spiritual connection.

Moving energy through breath has functioned as one of the primary healing processes in every ancient medical tradition. History proves we should pay attention to our breath to stay healthy.

BREATHING EXERCISES

The good news is you don't have to climb mountains to reap these benefits. You can practice them at your desk, at the airport, or even while in transit. Brief ten-minute breathing breaks throughout the workday are enough to help ward off work stress.

According to the American Institute of Stress, twenty to thirty minutes of slow breathing daily can reduce stress and anxiety (Ma et al. 2017). This doesn't need to be done all at once. Practicing throughout the day in small doses, like three ten-minute breathwork sessions, will have the same effect.

Relearning how to breathe slowly and deeply can take time. Start with five-minute breathing sessions and gradually build up the breathing practice time as your body acclimatizes. As with any exercise, check with your doctor before performing anything new. If you feel dizzy or lightheaded, stop the breathing exercise, stay seated, and return to breathing normally.

Get That App: *Many apps like Headspace, Breathe, Paced Breathing, and Calm have timed slow-paced breath cycles that promote better breathing.*

You can try several different breathing techniques to slow down breathing. Two of the breathing exercises I learned during my yoga training are explained below.

BOX BREATHING

Box breathing is an ayurvedic breathing practice popular among US Navy Seals for its calming effect. Tal Rabinowitz, founder and CEO of The DEN Meditation, explains in an online article, "It has incredibly ancient roots, with different techniques for calming, bringing in energy, refining focus, and relaxing the nervous system; however, the military popularized it and brought it mainstream" (Bunch 2021). Box breathing, as the name suggests, has equal inhalation and exhalation cycles, just like the four sides of a box. To practice box breathing:

- Sit comfortably in your chair or lie on the floor with your back on the mat.

- If sitting in a chair, place your feet on the floor hip distance apart.

- If lying on the floor, have your feet touching the floor and your knees bent.

- Lying on the floor is better for practicing box breathing because it minimizes the effects of gravity on your diaphragm.

- Breathe in, counting to four, slowly letting the air fill your lungs.

- Hold your breath for four counts or, if you have a timer visible, set it for four seconds.

- Slowly exhale through your mouth for four counts until you feel your naval touch your spine.

- Hold your breath for four counts.

- Repeat the above steps for five minutes.

ALTERNATE-NOSTRIL BREATHING

Alternate-nostril breathing is another yogic breathing exercise. In Sanskrit, it is called *nadi shodhana*. *Nadi* means "channel of flow," and *shodhana* means "purification." Here's how to practice:

- Sit in a comfortable upright posture with your head aligned over the spine and your shoulders relaxed by your side.

- Close your eyes or soften your gaze toward the floor.

- Close off your right nostril with your thumb. Inhale through your left nostril.

- Close off your left nostril with your pinky finger. Open the right nostril and exhale through it.

- Inhale through your right nostril. Close off your right nostril with your thumb.

- Open the left nostril and exhale. Inhale through your left nostril.

Slow breathing for five to ten minutes a day can significantly correct postural dysfunction, induce relaxation, and improve lung capacity (Russo, Santarelli, and O'Rourke 2017).

UPSHOT OF BREATH WORK

The upshot of slow breathing is that it elevates energy levels and increases your productivity. Shallow, hunched-over, rapid breathing doesn't just affect us physically but mentally as well. Overbreathing has its roots embedded in work stress, anxiety, and fear. These are the feelings that many of us are familiar with.

Posture Challenge: Practice slow breathing with awareness for just a few minutes daily. It can help you overcome these feelings of stress.

With this ancient tool, we can hack into our nervous system and attain a relaxed posture. I challenge you to carve out ten minutes in your day to practice slow breathing exercises.

CHAPTER 8

Relax

———

"Holding his leash is such a struggle," she said to her husband.

Lisa's right shoulder was sore, and walking her dog was becoming difficult. For the last three months, the pain had been progressively getting worst. Reaching forward would trigger a pain response. Even washing dishes was difficult.

Lisa is the CFO of a large hotel chain. She loves her job, but the last quarter had been stressful with financial constraints and the loss of a major hotel chain vendor. Her husband insisted she should go and get her arm checked.

Her doctor ordered an MRI, which showed no signs of fracture, and recommended she see a shoulder rehabilitation specialist. Over six weeks, I saw Lisa for soft tissue release around her shoulder and gave her a progressive strength training program. I educated her on pacing her work and using stress reduction techniques. At the intended conclusion of her posture coaching, Lisa was pain-free, but she enjoyed the program so much that she continued it for a year.

WORK STRESS

Close to 60 percent of computer office workers report shoulder and neck pain. Typical workloads add mental stress, which in turn leads to muscle pain. Eighty-three percent of US professionals suffer workplace stress, and US businesses lose up to $300 billion yearly because of it (Boyd 2011).

Work stress is the harmful physical and emotional response when work demands—like tight deadlines, staff shortages, and coworker relationships—exceed our resources. Work stress can manifest in many ways. Most noticeably, it can cause the onset of a physiological response resulting in musculoskeletal pain and poor posture.

SYMPATHETIC RESPONSE

We've all felt stress. No matter what the cause, physical or emotional, it sends the same pain signals. Stress adversely affects our nervous system and the way our nerves communicate. When stress levels are high, a signal travels from our brain to the nerves to protect us. Under this protection mechanism, our nerves stimulate our muscles to tighten and tense. Thus, stress can physically show itself in the form of muscle aches caused by this built-up muscle tension.

At the first encounter of significant stress, our body goes into survival mode. Unfortunately, our brain cannot differentiate between stress from a potential saber-toothed tiger or pressure from the increased number of projects at work. Our brain treats all stressors similarly and activates the fight-or-flight response, a natural reaction that helps us run or be ready to face danger. The physiologic response during fight-or-flight includes (Goldstein 2010):

- Rapid breathing

- Increased heart rate

- Increase in blood pressure

- Reduced blood flow

- Higher levels of cortisol, a stress hormone

- Tense muscles

The reduced blood flow to our muscles tightens them and raises their level of lactic acid. In turn, high lactic acid levels induce muscle soreness and send pain signals to our brains. This stress-to-pain cycle can continue in an endless loop for modern deskbound professionals.

THE POSTURAL STRESS RESPONSE

Dr. Erik Peper, a professor at San Francisco State University, has carried out a lot of research on how our modern work style affects our health. In one study, his team scrutinized deskbound office workers between the ages of seventeen and fifty-three using biofeedback devices that tracked shoulder and forearm muscle tension and monitored breathing rates (Peper 2003).

While typing at their average speed the office workers' heart rates were higher than normal, at ninety beats per minute, and their breathing rates doubled to twenty-four breaths per minute. Moreover: their neck muscle tension increased, and their skin became a better conductor of electricity, indicating high stress.

"What they were unaware about was the physiologic effects they were experiencing," he says in his YouTube interview with Inna Khazan, a faculty member at Harvard Medical School (Khazan 2020). While looking at her results, one of the study participants said, "I thought my shoulders were relaxed. I had no idea they were tight, and I was breathing so quickly."

Our static posture at the computer and repetitive typing action increases muscular tension. This tension, paired with an increased respiration rate, puts our body in an alarmed state—as if we are protecting ourselves from a threat.

THE STRESS CYCLE

The muscle tension we experience in our work environments is postural stress. Postural stress builds up by holding a prolonged static position, hunched over posture, and repetitive typing movements. This stress, as we have learned, causes pain.

All of our muscles like to go through a stress phase and a relaxation phase. When we want to move a part of the body, our brain sends a nerve signal to the muscles. The nerve signals cause our muscles to contract. Then the muscles relax until they are called upon to move again.

Postural Muscle Stress Cycle

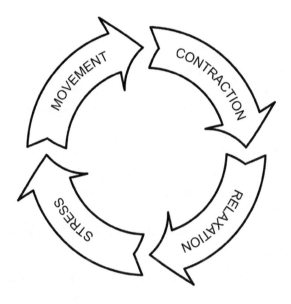

Caption: Postural Muscle Stress Cycle That's Incomplete in Office Workers

In the relaxation phase, our muscles regenerate. In the case of deskbound postures, our postural muscles stay active because we hold our body in a hunched position for extended periods. This causes muscles to become tight and rigid.

When we unplug and go home, these muscles should relax and return to their state of rest. But oftentimes, the muscle tension continues unless we take steps to actively relax them. The brain continues to signal the muscles to contract even when they are no longer needed for movement. This constant activation pattern leads to pain and injury. The longer you stay under stress, the poorer your posture and the more muscle pain you'll feel.

Physical stress isn't all that bad. We all need a healthy dose of physical stress in our lives. In fact, athletes intentionally use the muscle stress cycle to their advantage. They increase their training load to stress a given muscle and then follow it with a rest cycle.

But when physical stress becomes chronic, like in our everyday work environment, our muscles cannot regenerate.

Work Productivity Hack: *Taking short breaks to refresh throughout the day helps combat stress and increase productivity. Stepping away from the computer to change the scenery is important. Take your lunch break away from your desk. Even a five-minute break can help you recenter and reduce stress.*

As a deskbound professional, I used to endure a lot of stress—until the day I received a wake-up call from lower back pain. After a very long work project working extra hours at the office, my lower back pain got so bad that it became difficult to walk to the car. I wish I had known back then to pace myself and remove myself from work when I came home. I would have changed my work habits sooner if I had known rest and rejuvenation would help with pain, posture, and productivity.

Take it from me: you're more important than your job. Even when the projects become crucial and days get frantic. You don't have to compromise your health, and one way to prioritize being healthy is by being aware of the stress symptoms. Notice the effects of stress. Are your muscles tense? Are you breathing fast? Focus on the tension and breathing. Practicing awareness will help reduce the stress.

I practice the above awareness exercise with my clients regularly, and it helps them destress and relax. But some of my clients face a different significant challenge: their home is their workplace and disconnecting from work is difficult.

THE PANDEMIC SHIFT

During the pandemic, our homes transitioned into office spaces.

Diane, an executive assistant, came to me eight months into the pandemic with low back pain. "I know the couch might not be the best place to do my work. I have a workstation at home, but the kids kept interrupting me during my calls. It's just easier to work close to them," she said. She thought schools would open in the fall of 2020 and she just had to make things work until then.

The pressure of homeschooling her children while working as an executive assistant at a large healthcare company was making her sick. She was experiencing extreme pain. When I evaluated her posture, she had an anterior pelvic tilt—an extra arch in her lower back because of the way her body rested on the couch. The improper sitting position had compressed her spinal discs. Over the next three months, I worked with her on proper sitting technique, posture correction exercises, and stress management. Diane was pain-free and more productive at work after the program.

Working from home adds to the stress because the lines between work and personal life get blurred. On average, remote employees work three more hours per day (Davis 2020). If we total it up, that's fifteen extra work hours per week. As homes turn into offices, our always-on work culture has truly peaked. This is concerning for our health because that's fifteen more hours of constrained posture and work stress that leads to pain.

WAYS TO CURB WORK STRESS

Workplace stressors can wreak havoc on our health. We can take small steps to curb stress so it doesn't get in the way of our goals. Here are a few ways to combat work stress.

Identify Stressors: Reflecting on what's causing stress is the best way to identify the cause of your symptoms. List your biggest work priorities and how you handle them. Recording your priorities, thoughts, and actions will help you pinpoint the exact trigger. Once you know those stressors, you can find ways to navigate them differently or bring them up with your manager.

Exercise: Exercise is a stressbuster. Schedule short exercise breaks throughout the day to get a healthy dose of endorphins. Exercise circulates the blood to the brain, releases feel-good chemicals, and improves stress resilience.

Meditate: Meditation brings mental well-being. A few minutes of focusing on your breathing can help you relax and cope with stress by breaking your body's tension cycle. It enables you to stay calm and relaxed throughout the day. Start your day with a ten-minute meditation to set a relaxing tone. Taking short mindfulness breaks during the day is beneficial too. You can access my guided meditation to reduce work stress at this link www.aeshatahir.com/books.

Create Healthy Boundaries: It can be very tempting to feel the pressure to be available twenty-four hours a day. Hustle culture has made it seem like the norm to always be working. It's no wonder that this change in society has caused an increase in physical and mental maladies. Create healthy work boundaries for yourself by logging off work at six in the evening, blocking an hour for exercise, not checking emails at mealtime, and cultivating a healthy bedtime routine. Separating work from home will provide the necessary time to recharge.

Turn Off to Recharge: Make sure you switch off in the evening to avoid stress and burnout. Turning off means you step away from work entirely, not even thinking about it.

It's critical we take responsibility for our mental health. We can take these small steps to prioritize self-care and regenerate from work stress. Prioritizing our mental well-being is beneficial not only for us but also for everyone around us, including our families.

EMPLOYEE STRESS MANAGEMENT PROGRAMS

As individual employees take responsibility for their well-being, it's important to remember that organizations also need to shift the focus on stress reduction to change the wellness paradigm. The work environment is an essential factor in reducing chronic stress for employees. Less than half of US employees believe their organizations care about their work-life balance (APA 2013). This kind of imbalance can take a tremendous toll on our lives, causing 120,000 annual deaths (Boyd 2011). Its financial consequences are also staggering, costing US businesses $300 billion yearly.

To positively reshape workplace culture, employers should:

- Conduct regular employee stress screenings and recognize early stress symptoms

- Get to know their employees

- Provide training on effectively reducing stress to workplace leaders

- Set realistic goals and communicate clearly

- Provide mental health education programs on stress symptoms and their harmful effects

- Introduce postural health programs at work which emphasize the mental and physical health connection

One of the organizations that exemplify this company culture is PeopleG2. When employees cannot take a break from work stress, their productivity dips. Chris Dyer, the founder of the company, is a forward thinker and believes in prioritizing his team's wellness. He has created intentional processes signaling to employees it's okay to take time off to go on a vacation without being concerned about the workload they will have waiting when they return. "We implemented a program around vacation," he explains in our Zoom interview. "We asked our employees to set an out-of-office message which says the employee is on vacation and isn't going to read this email but instead delete it. When the employee returns from vacation, they send a screenshot or video recording of deleting all their unread emails."

PeopleG2 gave their employees the tools needed to say they are getting a complete break from work stress. Taking a dedicated block of personal time helps them recharge, connect with their family, and care for their mental health. This program has resulted in happy, healthy, and productive employees better equipped to contribute to the company's success. PeopleG2's approach reduced the cost of presenteeism. Presenteeism is when employees come to work but are disengaged due to stress.

UPSHOT OF RELAXATION

The upshot of taking time to relax is that we can break the chronic work-stress cycle. We can get out of the fight-or-flight mode and rejuvenate our muscles. In our modern work culture, we can work twenty-four hours a day, seven days a week, through different online platforms. In the short term, we might give in to the pressure, thinking nothing of it, but when work stress becomes chronic, it costs us our well-being.

Posture Challenge: I challenge you to step away from your desk station every thirty minutes. Take small breaks throughout the day and completely unplug at least one day of the week.

Relaxing and interrupting the chronic stress cycle will lead to a pain-free body and a relaxed mind.

CHAPTER 9

Posture for Empowerment

We all step into it in our unique way, and it exists within all of us. Many major organizations have a variety of traits and characteristics describing the skills needed for it.

It's leadership!

"Leadership" is a hot word these days. Good leadership skills are at the top of recruiters' competencies list when hiring or promoting people within an organization. Look up any executive-level role description, and you'll see communication, confidence, motivation, trustworthiness, and teamwork on top of the list. These leadership skills exist in each one of us, and you can hone them whether you are a project leader, an entrepreneur, or want to become a better leader in your personal life.

But what if our posture keeps us from showing our leadership ability and positively contributing to the workplace? Lack of appropriate leadership is a critical cause of workplace stress. In fact, over a third of American workers attribute workplace stress to inadequate leadership (Ferry 2018).

COMMUNICATION

Communication is the core leadership skill. It also comes at the top of the list of workplace stressors. In 2019, 80 percent of office workers correlated their stress to the poor communication practices of their leaders (First Up 2022). Having strong communication triples your effectiveness as a leader. When leading a team, good communication means clearly conveying your message and exuding confidence as a leader.

We can improve the delivery and perception of our message by adopting a positive posture. Our body posture during business meetings can radiate confidence and engagement. Ninety-three percent of all communication is nonverbal (Spence 2020). Seventy percent of the results of our interactions depend on how people feel about those encounters (Spence 2020). That means our body language plays a significant role in gaining favorable social results. Body posture also hints at our emotions, like anxiety and depression or confidence and calm. Actors and models get formal training to assume an upright posture for increased confidence and enhanced emotional communication.

Dr. Rob Holcroft attended drama school and worked as an actor and director with the Birmingham Royal Ballet and Hollywood before becoming a qualified physical therapist and psychotherapist. He specializes in posture and its effects on emotions. "I've been working with and studying the effects of posture for over twenty-three years. We all unwittingly sabotage our psychological and emotional well-being, as well as our physical health in the way that we sit, stand, and move, or more likely, don't move," he says, standing in front of the

TEDx audience and wearing a blue superman cape on his back and a yellow emblem on his chest (TEDx Talks 2017).

He explains how hunching over is perceived as a defeated and depressed position. People with emotional trauma might adopt a slouched position to protect their hearts, the center of their emotional energy. "Now, as a species, we sit [slouched] longer than ever. And I don't think it's a coincidence those suffering from mental health issues appear to be at an all-time high," he adds.

The toll a hunched-over posture takes on deskbound professionals' emotional health is rooted in our physiology and evolution. If we want to communicate effectively, having an upright posture signals to others that we are focused, calm, and confident.

CONFIDENCE

Our physiology dictates our confidence—an important leadership trait—through our posture. Sitting and standing in a slouched position can drive down our confidence.

A social scientist from the small Pennsylvanian town of Robesonia had self-doubt when she transferred to Princeton University to further her studies. Her life experience inspired her to be part of groundbreaking research on how posture impacts people's feelings, behaviors, and hormone levels. "I want to start by offering you a free no-tech life hack, and all it requires of you is this: that you change your posture for two minutes," she claims in a lively tone on the TED stage (Cuddy 2018). Dr. Amy Cuddy is a professor and researcher at

Harvard Business School, where she studies the psychological effects of body language.

"We know that our minds change our bodies but is it also true that our bodies change our minds?" she says, talking about the focus of her research.

Her work shows expansive postures with an open chest and head held high produce hormone levels promoting confidence. They found elevated testosterone, decreased cortisol, and dominant feelings of power in study participants with upright and expansive postures. It's not surprising hormonal levels in submissive body postures demonstrate the reverse.

"Here's what you get on cortisol. High-power [confident] people experience about a 25 percent decrease, and low-power people experience about a 15 percent increase. So, two minutes lead to these hormonal changes that configure your brain to be either assertive, confident, and comfortable, or stress-reactive, and, you know, feeling [sort of] shut down," she says, explaining the results of one of her studies. An unhunched posture is all about sparking the physiologic changes that will make us more confident.

Higher Confidence Hack: Next time you have a high-stakes situation or need extra confidence, stand tall in an expansive posture. An open and elevated pose, like hands reaching up to the ceiling or elbows fanning out by your side, will give you the hormonal boost to be confident.

Feelings of power and dominance in our upright and expansive posture correspond to primal animal behavior, in which alpha leaders have erect postures in the animal kingdom. Cognitive psychologists have concluded that proper posture can increase confidence and reduce stress. Assuming an unhunched posture aligns both our spine and our nervous system.

Professor Richard Petty, a cognitive psychologist from Ohio State University, says in his interview with *Fast Company* magazine that "we have all these associations" with height and power that "get triggered automatically when certain movements are made" (Giang 2015). He gives an example that if we put two people on a chair, one of them being higher than the other, the person on the higher chair will feel more confident and assertive. Sitting and standing in a tall and open posture signals our brain that we are powerful, which increases our confidence. He says, "The brain has an area that reflects confidence, but once that area is triggered, it doesn't matter exactly how it's triggered."

HIGHER SELF-WORTH AND SELF-ESTEEM

Leaders build strong teams at work using strong interpersonal skills, motivation, delegation, and problem-solving. Their ability to create high-functioning teams stems from their high self-esteem and belief in themselves.

Dr. Petty's team researched Ohio State students to find out whether an unhunched posture increases confidence in our abilities. In this study, they asked students to either sit up straight with an open chest or sit hunched over with their gaze down (Briñol, Petty, and Wagner 2009). The students then filled out a job application requiring them to list either three positive or negative personality traits that would contribute to their future job satisfaction and professional performance. Afterward, the students ranked themselves on how well they thought they would perform professionally in the future.

Dr. Petty's results showed that the way the students ranked themselves corresponded to their assumed posture. Students in unhunched postures believed in the positive traits they wrote on job applications, whereas those in a hunched-over stance didn't trust their ability to perform well. This suggests our posture impacts our beliefs and thoughts about our abilities. Upright position makes it easier to recognize our positive traits and empowers us with an optimistic belief in our abilities.

These findings are in congruence with Dr. Amy Cuddy's study of body language and its connection to leadership traits.

RESILIENCE TO STRESS

Another powerful leadership trait is resilience to stress. Team members expect their leaders to be calm and deliberate in their decisions and actions. They want leaders who aren't stress-reactive in high-stakes crises.

Dr. Nathan Considine, Dr. Elizabeth Broadbent, and their team at the University of Auckland have been interested in examining psychological distress as it relates to postural behavior (Nair et al. 2015). They experimented with deskbound professionals to determine if posture can positively affect their stress responses. They found when the participants with unhunched postures were presented with stressful situations, they had higher self-esteem, better moods, and less fear than hunched participants. This suggests that unhunched posture builds resilience to stress.

I want to invite you to try an experiment. Set a timer on your desk for four minutes. Now assume a slouched position in a chair and think of some negative experience for two minutes. After two minutes, switch to an upright position and hold the same negative thoughts. In which position could you keep your negative experience and self-sabotaging thoughts? Your answer might correlate with the experiments conducted by Dr. Peper.

Dr. Peper and his team report that 92 percent of deskbound professionals find it effortless to generate positive thoughts in an upright position (Wilson and Peper 2004). On the other hand, they find it easy to think of negative thoughts and memories in a slumped position.

Because muscular states can induce and regulate our emotional state, an upright posture is an important ingredient for confidence, higher self-esteem, less stress reactivity, and empowering thoughts and memories.

As a movement specialist, clients come to me for pain-free movement solutions. But an unexpected benefit of postural correction is the emotional empowerment my clients experience because the connection between muscular stress and emotional stress is robust.

Posture for Emotional Empowerment

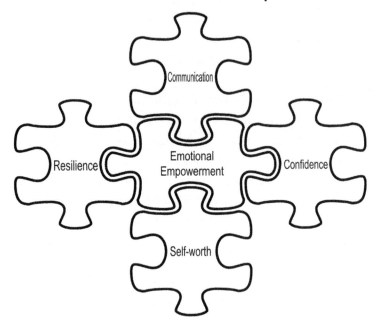

Caption: The Postural Empowerment Puzzle

UNLEASHING THE LEADER IN YOU

Work postures maintained for an extended time are associated with a high incidence of employee depression and anxiety.

"I used to love going to work, but I can't bring myself to go to work for the last two weeks," Jason told me during our initial screening. He is a thirty-two-year-old marketing director for a well-known pharmaceutical company with severe shoulder pain. His physician suggested seeing a posture coach.

While taking Jason's history, he told me he had skipped work for days because of nausea and vomiting related to workplace anxiety. This was his second round of a stress-induced digestive symptom episode. During the prior two months, his workload had increased manifold. In addition, he has been up for a promotion for the last two years, but at the yearly reviews, the executives told him he wasn't ready for the leadership role.

Jason has elevated, rounded shoulders. Elevated shoulders are the most common postural sign of stress. Next time you face a stressful situation, notice your shoulders. Most probably, they have climbed up to your ears. For deskbound professionals working in high-stress conditions, keeping the shoulders up due to work stress creates muscular recruitment patterns that lead to perpetual shoulder elevation.

We worked on Jason's elevated shoulders with a posture program that included breathing, stress management techniques, and corrective exercise. In twelve weeks, Jason's shoulders were back in place and pain-free. At his eight-week follow-up call, he told me about his promotion to the chief marketing officer position he had been striving for the last three years. As a coach, I'm always happy to see my clients live healthy lives, but watching them become empowered is an even more incredible privilege. And almost always, my clients' health and wellness are paired with career success.

Correcting our posture and living pain-free helps us step into greatness. The physiology of a better posture improves our beliefs about ourselves. It helps us realize that many things we have assumed about ourselves aren't true. There is no greater gift for us than self-love, self-acceptance, self-realization, and higher self-worth. An upright posture is an embodiment of creating a positive reality, vision, purpose, and ultimate success. It can carve us into the leaders we are meant to be.

STRESS AND EMOTIONAL WELL-BEING

As we have learned, stress, poor posture, and the inability to embrace leadership are very much linked. Unfortunately, stress, depression, and anxiety are a growing part of our lives today. Global statistics point to an increasing number of people struggling with mental health issues due to stress, and Americans are among the most stressed-out populations in the world. Fifty-five percent of Americans experience stress on any given day, which is 20 percent higher than the global average of 35 percent (Ray 2002).

Stress hits the working age group the hardest. In 2019, 94 percent of American workers experienced sustained workplace stress (Hansen 2021). Twenty-three percent of these workers ranked their stress levels high, and another 6 percent ranked their stress as unreasonably high. These numbers show the grim reality that work stress is more commonplace than we think. Fortunately, we live in a time when we talk more openly about our struggles than ever before.

Statistics reveal that heavy workloads, deadlines, and demanding leadership contribute to the problem. Stress due to work, if left untreated, can cause serious mental health problems. Our postural health is a tool that's easily accessible to all and can help us manage and limit the symptoms of stress while honoring our physiology. Along the way, we can embrace our inner leader.

INTEGRATING POSTURAL EMPOWERMENT

With so much research and data pointing to the connection between posture and our emotional health, here are a few tips to take care of yourself throughout the workday.

Embrace Power Poses: Power poses throughout the day can help fight negative emotions. Set a timer or place Post-it Notes around your desk as reminders to practice open and tall posture for two-minute intervals throughout the workday. You are changing the chemistry in your brain to encourage you. Make power posing a priority before any critical high-risk situation like an organizational meeting, job interviews, and filling out job applications.

Unhunch Your Confidence: Sit and stand in an upright posture with shoulders down, chest wide open, head over the spine and gaze straight up throughout the day—especially when you experience self-doubt and negative thoughts. Instead of validating those thoughts by hunching, try to look up, sit tall, and ward off those thoughts with upright physiology.

Look Up to Level Up Your Thoughts: Position your monitor an inch or two above your eye level so you can sit tall in your chair. In the car, adjust your rear-view mirror slightly higher so that you drive in an unhunched position. A tall posture will help you feel taller, too, triggering your power hormones and empowering you to become a confident and self-assured leader.

EMOTIONAL HEALTH OF ORGANIZATIONS

It's noteworthy that workplace stress isn't detrimental to only workers' health. It impacts the health of companies as well. Stress, anxiety, and depression cost the global economy around one trillion in lost productivity. In the US, depression costs fifty-one billion due to absenteeism from work and twenty-six billion in healthcare costs (Health 2022). The compromised mental well-being of the workforce is a health and financial epidemic.

A workspace equipped with resilient, poised leaders creates an environment and a team that works in harmony to produce better work with less stress. Providing posture correction training as part of leadership development at your organization is critical to helping fill the gap of resilient and confident leadership. When this gap is filled, it will lead to higher productivity, lower healthcare costs, and a happier workforce.

UPSHOT OF POSTURE FOR EMPOWERMENT

The upshot of having a better posture is it can induce and regulate a more positive emotional state. An upright posture is an ingredient for self-confidence, higher self-esteem, less stress reactivity, and access to empowering thoughts and memories.

Posture Challenge: Fix your posture to hone the necessary leadership skills. From communicating to building trust, you can strengthen each one of the leadership skills with better posture.

The growing pattern of emotional health issues in our population will not end if we don't promote posture programs at work.

CHAPTER 10

Activity—The Antidote To the Sitting Disease

Lack of activity destroys the good condition of every human being, while movement and methodical physical exercise save it and preserve it.

—PLATO.

Melanie Archer received a promotion to a loan officer after years of being a bank teller. She liked her new cubicle and sitting in a comfortable chair after standing all day for three years. But after a year in her new position, she began to have issues with her back. She went to see her primary care physician for lower back pain, which would worsen when she tried to bend. "I'm unable to bend and lift my two-year-old toddler," she explained. "Pick-ups and drop-offs at the daycare are very hard."

The doctor prescribed her an over-the-counter painkiller and suggested she start exercising.

Melanie had a pronounced lower back arch with weak core muscles. She wasn't thrilled about the recent loss of tone around her waistline and the ten-pound weight gain. "I eat a healthy diet. I haven't made any drastic changes in my lifestyle. I'm not sure what's going on," she told me.

I explained to Melanie how working as a teller meant she was standing and moving most of the time. Her body was active in that position. Inactivity, along with slumping in her chair, had weakened her core muscles and reduced calorie expenditure. Her weak core muscles were the root cause of the pain.

Over the next six weeks with me, she strengthened her core, stabilizing muscles and glutes, and stretched her tight muscles. Along with that, she requested frequent movement breaks from her manager. After twelve weeks of training, Melanie was back to being pain-free.

ENDLESS SITTING

What's alarming about Melanie's story is the outsize impact of a sedentary workstyle on her health in a very short period. It's also shocking to see the transition of humans from an active leg-based species to a completely automated and sedentary one in just over a century.

Keith Diaz, an exercise physiologist and assistant professor of behavioral medicine at Columbia University Medical Center, has been looking into the sedentary behaviors of American workers (Davis 2019). For one study, he analyzed the physical activity of over seven thousand adults older than forty-five for four years. These adults wore a hip-mounted accelerometer, an electromechanical device to measure acceleration forces. The results showed sedentary behavior, on average, accounted for about 12.3 hours of an average sixteen-hour waking day (CNN 2017).

Many deskbound clients aren't aware of the cost of physical inactivity, but sedentary behavior and postural problems are the cause of many pain issues that my clients face.

THE POSTURE AND SITTING CONNECTION

Sedentary behavior contributes to poor posture, creating body stress and straining our muscles. Hours of sitting tighten up our leg muscles from a combination of inactivity and constant bending of our hip and knee joints. This continuous muscle tension builds painful knots in our body called trigger points. Trigger points are specific muscle areas that are sore to touch. These tighter muscles can throw off our gait and balance.

This innocently relaxed position also takes a tremendous toll on our spine. The seated position loads the weight of our upper body onto our lower back. Added pressure on the lower back vertebrae compresses them. Just like placing a brick on a marshmallow tower, our vertebrae collapse under pressure. The seated position puts 90 percent more pressure on our lower back than standing and walking (Williams 2021). On the other hand, the standing position distributes our body weight evenly throughout the spine, hips, knees, and ankles. Extended periods of sitting are behind the increased occurrence of lower back pain in office workers.

As the work stress builds up during the day, our bodies start slouching. Our chins drop to the chest, and our shoulders become rounded and climb up to our ears. Droopy shoulders increase the pressure on our cervical spine, leading to a distorted neck curve and increasing the effect of gravitational forces on our head, neck, and shoulders. This pressure builds over time, leading to neck pain, decreased shoulder mobility, shoulder pain, and headaches.

FROM MUSCLES TO METABOLISM

An extended seated posture not only stresses our spine but also weakens the muscles. Prolonged sitting shuts down the activity of our leg muscles. Do your legs feel sluggish and heavy after a long sitting session? If they do, you're experiencing a side effect of sedentary behavior. Prolonged sitting makes our calf muscles weak and strained. Calf muscles are known as the second heart because they help pump blood up toward our heart, working against gravity.

But weak calf muscles are less able to return the blood to our hearts. "Sitting shuts down electrical activity in the legs," says Dr. Toni Yancey, professor of health services at UCLA's Fielding School of Public Health. "Sitting makes the body less sensitive to insulin, causes calorie-burning to plummet, and slows the breakdown of dangerous blood fats, lowering the 'good' HDL cholesterol" (Fiorenzi 2018).

The reduced blood flow causes the slowing down of cholesterol and fat molecules from arteries to muscles. This results in the deposit of cholesterol on arterial walls. Cholesterol is a waxlike substance in our blood, and too much of it can be harmful. In fact, high cholesterol levels are a risk factor for cardiovascular disease and stroke. Sitting also drops the level of the enzyme that turns harmful LDL cholesterol into good HDL cholesterol by 95 percent (Nazario 2021).

Sitting also impedes the blood flow to our digestive organs, like the stomach and intestines. This position compresses all the organs in our midsection, reducing the gastrointestinal muscles' peristalsis (wavelike movements of the stomach). Oftentimes, slumped sitting episodes are responsible for digestive issues like acid reflux, gas, bloating, and constipation.

Our metabolism slows considerably when constantly sitting during the workday because the breakdown of fats and sugars is also blocked. Gavin Bradley, director of Active Working, an international group aimed at reducing excessive sitting, explains, "Metabolism slows down 90 percent after thirty minutes of sitting. And after two hours, good cholesterol drops 20 percent" (Schulte 2015).

Compromised circulation, squeezing of the gastrointestinal tract, and slow metabolism are linked to hunched posture and poor muscle activation. However, indirectly, poor posture nevertheless increases the risk of premature death due to metabolic diseases.

My college friend Connor, a computer software engineer, was delighted when he landed a job with a big tech firm. "It's a 100 percent remote job. I'm wildly excited," he told me on the phone after accepting the job.

Connor is an ex-collegiate runner, so I call him occasionally to ask running questions. One day he said, "I'm a bit stressed out these days. My cholesterol is high, and my ankles often swell." At the time of this conversation, he was three years into his remote position. "You know, I've done this to myself. I need to make some serious lifestyle changes. Doc says I am at a higher risk for heart disease," he lamented. He was working long and unstructured hours, and after work, he would play console games with his coworkers as part of a Discord league.

I was just shocked at the news. *No way*, I thought. *My friend, who's only thirty-eight, a collegiate runner, and someone who exercises every day, can't be having that issue.*

But much of the US workforce is in the same boat as Connor. More than 80 percent of jobs in the US are sedentary (Church et al. 2011). Cardiovascular disease-related mortality rates are on the rise in working-age Americans (Curtin 2019), and there are 3.2 million premature deaths yearly due to a sedentary lifestyle (World Health Organization 2022).

MOVE, MOVE, MOVE

Despite their efforts, people who exercise an hour a day are at the same risk of medical issues related to a sedentary lifestyle. Katy Bowman, a movement specialist, writes in her book *Move Your DNA: Restore Your Health Through Natural Movement* that "Active sedentary is a new category of people who are fit for one hour but sitting around the rest of the day, you can't offset ten hours of stillness with one hour of exercise" (Bowman 2014).

The common belief that working out one hour a day will improve our health doesn't hold true anymore. Just like we can't ace a test by studying for only fifteen minutes a day during the semester, you can't outrun a sedentary lifestyle with an hour of workout. Some of my most intellectually fit friends think they can shake off twelve hours of sitting with an hour of exercise. But the verdict is in: it's about moving our bodies frequently and in various ways.

It's best to take a movement break every thirty minutes. This break can be walking around, light stretching, or following along with a ten-minute workout video. Even a three-minute movement break every thirty minutes can combat the effects of sitting, like reduced blood sugar and harmful cholesterol levels (Smith et al. 2021). The more you move, the better your posture and overall health.

And wait! Don't cancel your gym membership just yet. Sedentary workers who do take that hour to exercise indeed have a lower risk of disease than their completely inactive counterparts. Exercise alone might not be enough to combat the risk of prolonged sitting during the day, but it still has worthwhile health benefits.

STAND MORE AT WORK

I see many postural clients with metabolic diseases like high cholesterol, cardiovascular issues, and obesity. Better work habits—switching between sitting and standing positions—are part of my posture treatment protocol. Many of my clients have shared concerns about position changes disrupting their work and decreasing their focus. But the reality is quite the opposite.

Researchers report a 65 percent boost in productivity at a call center after a standing desk intervention (Edwardson et al. 2018). Alternating sitting and standing intervals enhance job performance and work engagement and lower occupational fatigue and absenteeism.

Investing in an adjustable desk or desk attachment is an easy way to engage our lower leg muscles, increase our blood circulation, and improve oxygen concentration in our bloodstream—leading to improved focus, memory, and productivity. Standing activates a different part of our brain than sitting, advancing our focus and problem-solving ability. It also lowers our cholesterol and trims our waistline by burning 0.15 kcal more per minute than sitting (Saeidifard et al. 2018). This extra calorie loss can add up to a twenty-pound loss over five years by just using a standing desk.

Alternating between sitting and standing positions adjusts the load on the joints and reduces the stiffness of muscles. The flexibility of an adjustable height desk brings a welcome relief from neck, shoulder, and back pain. Pain relief is sure to improve focus and productivity.

It's easy to develop the habit of standing at work by starting with small intervals. But like any new behavior, it can take time to acclimatize. Start by standing for ten minutes every hour and increase the time by five minutes every week. Setting a timer on your phone as a reminder makes it easy to remember to switch positions.

Overall, alternating our work positions increases energy, improves posture, and reduces fatigue levels and the risk of injury from being static all day.

COMBATING THE SEDENTARY LIFESTYLE

While being tied to the computer all day may be inevitable, we can infuse more activity into our day. After being diagnosed with lower back pain, I started changing my work routine to incorporate more movement. I recommend the same small habits to my clients. Below are some of the changes that go beyond movement breaks and standing desks.

Keep Movement Equipment Handy: Making movement a priority is easy if it becomes a natural part of your day. Wear comfortable shoes to work so you can walk often. Keep some essential exercise equipment close to your workstation, like a set of moderate-effort dumbbells, a tube resistance band, and a foam roller. You'll be more likely to use the equipment if you see it.

Download that App: You can download many apps on your phone or computer for a reminder to get up and do different movements like squats, lunges, and going up the stairs. You can set them up with your movement preferences too. Some of the available apps are Move, StandUp, and PC WorkBreak.

Rethink Your Meetings: Meetings are a perfect time to move *and* get work done. Try to turn your brainstorming sessions or in-person calls into walking meetings. Walking meetings help increase creativity and focus. Consider proposing walking meetings to your manager and HR team—they might be impressed by your knowledge and commitment to wellness.

Combating a sedentary occupational style can feel challenging, but making small workday changes can lead to big health rewards. The key is to make movement easy and natural.

A CASE FOR WELLNESS PROGRAMS AT WORK

Many organizations recognize the benefits of exercise programs to their employees and the company's bottom line. They are investing in a culture of wellness that leads to the happiness, safety, and productivity of the workforce. But there is still much work to do.

Companies prioritizing wellness can build trust with their employees, leading to employee retention and the hiring of top talent. Above all, recognizing that a human with physical and mental needs is on the other end of the computer screen is a solid reason to have wellness programs at work. Programs that include movement interventions during the workday and exercise opportunities ultimately increase employee engagement and productivity.

IKEA in Glasgow is one such business. "A healthy work environment is a priority in its own right in IKEA's UK business plan," says Jill Burgess, the store's human resource manager (Maxwell 2008).

This store is leading the way in employee health by providing their employees with podiatric care, fitness classes, and massage services for free as part of their health promotion program. At first, many employees just tried the services out of curiosity for the innovative idea. Soon, though, they noticed the health benefits of these services.

One floor associate shares, "It's a good perk. IKEA is obviously interested in the well-being of staff and is very people-oriented." IKEA also recently added a Fit for Work week to their health promotion program, offering various fitness activities during that week, and the staff likes to participate regularly.

As a result, IKEA Glasgow has higher-than-average employee retention, frequent employee referrals, and far lower absenteeism when compared with other companies in the same industry.

Other organizations can follow the example set by IKEA Glasgow if they want higher productivity, boosted bottom lines, lower healthcare costs, and improved employee retention.

UPSHOT OF ACTIVITY

The upshot of activity is it relieves pressure on our lower back and increases blood circulation. A sitting lifestyle is costing us our health. The scientifically proven reality is that a minimum amount of exercise will not reverse the harmful effects of prolonged sitting.

Posture Challenge: Aim to transition at least one meeting during the week to a walking meeting either on the phone or in-person. Taking small steps to incorporate regular movement in various forms helps combat the adverse health effects of sitting in a slumped position.

PART 3

CORRECTIVE
EXERCISE

Setting Up a Desk Station

We are on the last and most important component of our BRACE model: corrective exercise. In this part of the book, I'll introduce you to many postural exercises you can do from the comfort of your office space throughout the day. Most of the exercises use common office props like your desk, chair, or the wall. You can incorporate a resistance band, dumbbells, yoga mat, and foam roller for some exercises to support your workout.

The good news is you don't need the cable pulley system and squat rack for a posture workout. You can create the ideal space to build and maintain your natural posture with just a few essential pieces. When setting up an office gym, I like to improvise. You'll see a lot of easy everyday swaps in the following list.

EQUIPMENT

Here are a few pieces of equipment needed for the postural exercise program in the following few chapters.

Yoga Mat: A yoga mat is the most basic and used workout equipment providing support for exercises performed on the floor. It provides cushioning on hard surfaces and a grip for hands and feet. You can always use a couple of towels instead, especially if you're traveling and you don't have access to a mat.

Foam Roller: This postural exercise program incorporates self-massage to release muscle tension. It's an excellent way for people of all fitness abilities to pinpoint tight areas with adhesions in their muscles and treat them by applying direct pressure. There are different foam rollers depending on the pressure you want to apply: soft, firm, and rigid. I recommend starting with a soft foam roller and progressing as you feel you can use more pressure. Foam rolling is great for improving muscular balance, and helps ensure the opposing muscles are equally strong, have better flexibility, better movement, and have less risk of pain.

Lacrosse Ball: The lacrosse ball is another inexpensive and highly portable massage tool that releases tight spots for desk jockeys like us. It helps relieve pain and improve the function of our muscles. Honestly, it doesn't always feel good to work with the lacrosse ball at first. The first time I tried it, I couldn't handle the pain of breaking adhesions. You will feel better the more you use it. You can also use a softer tennis ball that applies less pressure and can help repair and prevent the misalignment of tight and weak muscles.

Resistance Bands: Resistance bands are thick rubber bands that come in color-coded resistance levels. These bands are a great way to add resistance for building strength. These bands can help with muscle activation and increase our range of motion. For example, placing the band around your legs during squats activates your hip abductors. Having two to three bands of different resistance levels is a good idea. A tube resistance band that you can tie around your legs would also work.

Dumbbells: Dumbbells are a staple of any strength workout. They are versatile and you can use them in any bodyweight exercise. Smaller dumbbells are great for postural exercises. I recommend my clients have two sets, one small and one medium. A light weight would be somewhere between two and five pounds, and a medium weight can be between eight and fifteen pounds. If you're new to exercising, stick with a lighter set of weights for the first eight to twelve weeks of the program until you feel comfortable progressing. You can also use two full water bottles instead of dumbbells at any time.

This list consists of the most essential desk workout items. With these items in your office gym, you can do all the postural exercises in this book easily on your own time.

LISTEN TO YOUR BODY

Our body tells us how it feels and what it would like. Listen to your body while implementing this exercise program. Relax your body while exercising, and only perform the exercises you are physically comfortable with. These simple exercises are easy on your body but, when done regularly, have a significant impact on your posture.

It's best to consult your physician before starting a new exercise program. If these exercises cause you any discomfort, discontinue. You should visit a physical therapist or a physician for further insight if you experience discomfort or pain while performing these exercises. When working out, it is essential to warm up with a five-minute walk or march in place.

EXERCISE VIDEO LIBRARY

I've created a video library of all the postural exercises in this book and some bonus exercises which are not in this book. These videos demonstrate the proper form and the equipment required for these exercises. You can find them at www.aeshatahir.com/books.

CHAPTER 11

Symmetry Matters

——

"The planets, moons, and stars exhibit symmetry widely," said the voice over the speakers

I was taking in the beauty of the night sky and basking in the Milky Way's glory. Watching this display of pervasive universal symmetry at the Hayden Planetarium in NYC was striking.

Some people might say asymmetry is the reason for life in the universe: the wild card that leads to change. I disagree.

I belong to the camp of scientists who study the symmetry of the universe. Blame it on my perfectionist mindset, but I use mathematical equations to show that balance is more pervasive than asymmetry. Planets and stars are symmetric due to the force of gravity, and this symmetric force applies to more than just cosmic objects.

Symmetry is omnipresent. From snowflakes to sunflowers, spider webs to starfish: symmetry is everywhere. Humans desire symmetry, from hanging pictures straight on the wall to straight eyeliner while applying makeup. This desire for symmetry even impacts what we find attractive. Our skeletal and muscular systems crave symmetric balance too.

The human body exhibits symmetry. Our body parts, including muscles, are symmetrical along a plane running from head to toe. This balance of body structures results in balanced physical functions.

SYMMETRIC HUMAN BODY

The simplest movements in the human body require a complex interplay of many skeletal structures while keeping our body stable under the external load. The structural symmetry of the human movement system allows posture to be balanced relative to our center of gravity (Lu and Chang 2012).

We look at two common forms of symmetry in relation to our posture. Bilateral symmetry, which is the balance between the right and left sides of the body, allows the skeleton's natural alignment. The second type of symmetry relates to the muscles in the front and back of our bodies. Imagine a sheet of glass dividing our bodies laterally into two halves. The distribution of muscle strength on both sides of the body dictates our posture.

Many life factors can lead to asymmetry. Dr. Kyle Stull, professor of exercise science at Concordia University and content manager for the National Academy of Sports Medicine, explained during our Zoom interview, "Asymmetries come from favoring one side or an injury on one side which we think has [been] rehabilitated, but it hasn't. These asymmetries give rise to poor posture."

Repetitive stress, sports, ergonomics, movement habits, body weight, and pregnancy can cause an asymmetrical skeleton. According to Dr. Stull, "Muscle imbalances are the result of adaptations. As humans, we're wonderful adapters. Whatever position we stay in, our body will adapt to that."

Deskbound professionals use the mouse with a preferred arm and lean over their desks using the front side of their bodies. Sometimes they sit on a preferred leg and stand with weight on a preferred side. "Due to poor posture or dominance or injury, one muscle starts pulling on the joint more than the opposing muscle. That is muscle imbalance. And it is the result of just adaptation over time," says Dr. Stull.

These asymmetric movement patterns cause muscular imbalances, disrupting the normal functioning of a body designed to perform within a symmetric paradigm.

MUSCULAR IMBALANCE

Offsets in strength and function between the two opposing muscle groups lead to painful movement. When building a house, the weight of the building must be distributed evenly. If the foundation isn't placed symmetrically, the frame will collapse from uneven pressure distribution. Similarly, our joint movements depend on our muscles having symmetrical strength. Our body's design needs equal load distribution throughout the skeleton to properly function without pain.

Dr. Vladimir Janda was a pioneer in the assessment of musculoskeletal pain. As a physician at the Department of Rehabilitation at Charles University in Prague, he studied muscle function in the locomotor system. His research found that muscle imbalance occurs when some muscle groups become inhibited and weak while others become tight and overactive. The balance of muscle length and strength is lost, which brings on changes in tissues, such as inflammation and pain. These tissue changes impact our movement while doing daily chores, lending our whole body to adapt to the imbalance. So, for best functionality, our body needs a balance of muscle flexibility and strength between opposing muscles surrounding the joints.

THE IMBALANCE CHAIN REACTION

Janda classified muscles throughout the body into two groups based on their function: mobilizer and stabilizer muscles (Comerford and Mottram 2001).

Mobilizer muscles are responsible for performing active movements in joints. These muscles are primarily visible and placed superficially under our skin. They tend to tighten with repeated and extended activity. The dominant mobilizers for slouched office workers are the chest muscles, hip flexors, front thigh muscles, and inner thigh muscles.

Then we have the stabilizer muscles. These muscles lie opposite to mobilizers and are embedded deep inside our bodies. They are available on demand but don't automatically fire upon movement because they don't actively fight the force of gravity. When the mobilizers take over the bulk of work, the stabilizers become weak and lengthened. They lose their tone and become soft over time. Abdominal muscles and gluteal muscles are perfect examples of weak stabilizer muscles in office workers. While sitting in a chair, we aren't using the correct muscles to retain our stability. These muscles require daily activation in varying forms to keep them toned and firm.

A chain reaction of imbalance starts in which some muscles are incredibly tight and can't sustain more work while others are weak and unable to function. Dr. Phil Page, Scrape cofounder and instructor and an athletic trainer for major American sports teams says in an article that "Changes within one part of the system will cause the body to attempt homeostasis [balance], resulting in compensations or adaptations elsewhere within the system" (Moore 2020). The risk of injury increases 2.6 times if muscular balance deviates more than 15 percent from the typical functional balance (Knapik et al. 1992).

BUT AREN'T WE ASYMMETRIC?

Though our body works as a complete unit, some organs and body parts aren't symmetric. As my friend says, "We all have asymmetries." Some asymmetry is normal.

This bears repeating: Some asymmetry is normal.

Our heart lies on the left, and the liver on the right. One lung is bigger than the other, and our diaphragm is also bigger on one side, so we breathe fuller on one side. Most of us have a dominant arm, which affects our shoulder's elevation. One leg is better at static balancing, while the other is better at motion.

Slight asymmetry has no adverse consequences.

With over a decade of experience as a movement specialist, I have yet to see someone who doesn't have slight asymmetries. Heck, even I have them. The key is to pay attention to the ones that cause harm. If the movement causes pain and the body's functionality reduces, the asymmetry is harmful. Injuries occur when this dominance goes too far, and we lose proper functioning on one side of our body. When I work with my clients, I evaluate how they generally move and how long they have experienced discomfort. I then focus on correct movement patterns and workday habits for a healthy movement pattern.

HOW ASYMMETRIC ARE YOU?

Our posture is related to how balanced our body is. This body balance helps us control the movement of our muscles by defining where we are in space, a concept called neuromuscular proprioception. This sensory system in our body determines where and how our body moves at conscious and subconscious levels. Inflammation and injury to muscles containing these proprioceptors lead to loss of control, which we call instability, and can increase our risk of falls.

Awareness of our asymmetry is the first step toward improving muscle imbalance and posture. A single leg balance test can create a baseline for our lower body muscle asymmetry (Physiopedia, 2023). This test is carried out on a single leg without shoes or socks and with the hands placed on the hips so they are not used for support.

Only perform this test while standing beside a wall or with someone who can hold you if you lose balance. If you are not sure about your balance, taking the test with a movement specialist is best to prevent a fall.

The steps for the single-leg balance test are as follows.

- Take your shoes off, keep your eyes open, place your hands on your hip bones, and stand on one leg.

- Start a timer as soon as your second foot leaves the ground.

- Stop the timer when the second foot touches the ground again or the hands reach for support.

- If you can stand on both legs without losing balance for the same amount of time, then your body has bilateral symmetry.

- The leg you can stand on longer is your balancing leg, and the other leg is your mobilizing leg. Usually, this is on the dominant side of your body.

- If you cannot stand for ten seconds or less, you are at a greater risk of injury from a fall.

In fact, the inability to hold a single leg stance for ten seconds in middle-aged and older adults doubles the risk of death from any cause (Araujo et al. 2022).

If you want to challenge yourself further, repeat the test for the longest interval you can balance on each leg and repeat with your eyes closed. You will be surprised how quickly you fall when your eyes are closed. Here are the targets that different age groups should be able to manage (Mosley 2022):

- Under 40: 45 seconds with eyes open, 15 seconds with eyes closed

- Aged 40–49: 42 seconds open, 13 seconds closed

- Aged 50–59: 41 seconds open, 8 seconds closed

- Aged 60–69: 32 seconds open, 4 seconds closed

- Aged 70–79: 22 seconds open, 3 seconds closed

Anything below these target times means you have muscle imbalances that reduce your flexibility and proprioception.

UP AND DOWN THE CHAIN

Different segments of the body allow movement at a joint.

When my boys were toddlers, we danced to "Dem Bones" by James Weldon Johnson. Because the song describes how our body parts work together, my kids used to touch all their body parts while we wiggled and danced to the music. This interconnected chain of the body is called the kinetic chain. Dr. Arthur Steindler, who originated this concept, described the muscles, bones, ligaments, tendons, joints, and neurologic input systems as the main structures of the chain (Smidt

1994). The force transference occurs from the nervous system to the musculoskeletal system for movement to occur. Dr. Stull explained it to me this way: "We have a layer of muscles and other types of connective tissues that connect from our eyebrows, goes over the top of our head, all the way down our spine, and to our toes."

Our posture is the alignment of the interconnected segments in our kinetic chain. Misalignment at one of the segments affects the other elements up and down the kinetic chain. "So, think about altering the length and tension [strength and flexibility balance] in the connective tissues up here in our head. That alteration is going to have a direct impact on our lower body mechanics," says Dr. Stull. How we sit, stand, and work influences not just one body part but the rest of the body too. Muscle imbalance at our shoulder joint can travel to the hip, knee, ankle, and connected muscles.

Valerie, a computer programmer, took up running eight weeks prior to when she came to see me in August 2019. She had a dull ache at the front side of her left hip. It would travel down her outer thigh during and after her run. For work, she would sit at her desk for an average of ten hours a day while coding for a well-known media company.

Her standing and squatting postural assessment revealed a hip hike on her left side and shoulder elevation on her right. Further evaluation of daily functional activities showed that she had a habit of standing and sitting on her left side. Our muscle-brain connection gets us into the habit of using one side of the body or specific muscles. For Valerie, her neuro-muscular pattern was to favor her left leg.

Her right shoulder was higher than her left shoulder due to this hip hike. Both her shoulder muscle dysfunction and hip dysfunction are related to each other. Just like a train has compartments, our body parts are our body's compartments linked to each other. A single weak link can make the whole train run off track.

I worked on correcting her muscle imbalances by strengthening the weak muscles and stretching the tight muscles on both sides of her body. In ten weeks, she was pain-free.

LET'S GET EVEN

Small, unhealthy habits can create muscle imbalances. These habits might include picking up groceries only on one side, sitting cross-legged, or kicking the ball with just one leg.

Avoid the Lean: Keep your body as straight as possible, balancing the weight evenly on both feet. Most of us stand with weight on one side, keeping a soft bend in the other knee. I see many clients who could avoid muscle imbalances by evenly distributing their body weight from side to side and front to back.

Modify Repetitive Tasks: Alternate computer tasks with attending meetings. If you frequently use the same side to talk on the phone, use a headset or put the phone on speaker.

Wear Even Shoes: Wear comfortable shoes without a heel lift. Even sneakers can have lifted heels. It's best to wear shoes with equal padding under the toes and heels. This is called the shoe's offset. You can ask a shoe store associate about it next time you shop. Avoid wearing high heels, which can affect the body's center of gravity and the muscle balance of your lower legs.

Switch the Bed Side: You have probably been sleeping on the same side of the bed for years. Every morning you wake up, you put the same foot down on the floor and reach with the same arm for the alarm clock. Continuing this pattern on autopilot helps you keep your routine but wreaks havoc on your muscle balance. Try to switch the side of the bed you sleep on every three to four weeks.

Walk Laterally: Try walking sideways during your movement break for a few minutes daily. Make sure you move both to the right and the left.

UPSHOT OF SYMMETRY

The upshot of symmetry is that using both sides of our body and evenly distributing the weight over our feet leads to a balanced posture. Symmetry is a universal phenomenon that applies to our bodies the same way it does to planets. We develop muscle imbalances due to repetitive typing, reclined positions, and lack of movement. These imbalances can cause inefficient neuromuscular habits and painful movement.

Posture Challenge: Try using your nondominant side to brush your teeth, reach for the plate, and go down the steps. Frequently switching up which side you use will keep your brain guessing and strengthen your proprioception and muscle balance.

We can attain functional symmetry when our body's muscles work together with equal strength. Simple changes in daily habits can prevent muscle imbalances and help us regain our natural posture.

CHAPTER 12

iPosture

Legend has it that Zeus doomed the Titan Atlas to carry the heavens upon his shoulders. "Atlas, under strong constraint, holds up the broad sky with his head and tireless hands, standing at the ends of the earth," writes Hesiod in the *Theogony* (Hesiod 1997).

Many artworks show Atlas hunched over, laboring under the weight with a forward head, bent neck, chin dropped to his chest, and shoulders caved in.

Walk into an office building, and you'll see the same posture in deskbound workers with their rounded shoulders, heads hanging in front, and round upper spines. It looks as if they are carrying the weight of the world on their shoulders.

UPPER BODY iPOSTURE

In today's technological age, people under the high demands of work are literally carrying extra weight on their shoulders, not only metaphorically. iPosture is the modern posture assumed while using computers and phones. Slumped shoulders, eyes looking down, and a compressed back are the primary characteristics of this posture.

It puts a hefty load on our spine and muscles due to the heavy head we carry up above. The human head weighs twelve pounds, close to the size of a bowling ball, and accounts for approximately 8 percent of our body mass (Gekhman 2006).

Human brains are larger than other primate brains. On the one hand: this gives us extraordinary brainpower. On the other: when we're slouched, it causes headaches, jaw pain, neck pain, and shoulder pain.

Seven vertebrae and twenty muscles in our neck support our head. In a neutral position, our head exerts force straight down the spine, and its weight is balanced evenly (Eidelson 2019). The problem occurs when we tilt our head forward. In this case, the downward force on the spine increases to thirty-two pounds at two inches titled forward and forty-two pounds at three inches (Hansraj 2014).

Sustaining this pressure is a lot to ask from our small neck muscles and can often cause pain and fatigue. This tilt also goes by the name "text neck," based on the common forward protruding of our head while using cell phones for texting.

Our neck and shoulder regions are a hub for many nerves exiting and entering the brain and spine. This is why hunched posture often leads to nerve compression, which in turn can cause numbing of the hands and arms. "In a hunched posture, we already have a system that's stretched and weak.

Add the weight of the head and you can easily add in the nerve compression due to pressure. Now it's a triple situation that can compromise nerve health. Many of the nerves are starting from the spine, exiting the spine, traveling through the shoulder girdle and into the arms," said Dr. Shelly Karbowski during our Zoom interview. Dr. Karbowski has more than thirty years of experience in physical therapy and is the founder and operator of TruWell Physical Therapy in Commerce, Michigan.

How Heavy Is Your Head?

12 lbs. (5.4 kg) 32 lbs. (15 kg) 42 lbs. (19 kg)

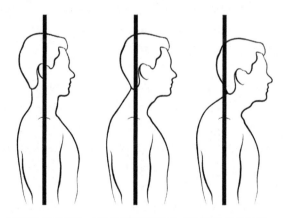

NORMAL POSTURE   2 IN (5 CM) FORWARD   3 IN (8 CM) FORWARD

42 lbs Head

Every inch of forward head posture can increase the head's weight on the spine by an additional ten pounds (or 4.5 kg).

Caption: Pressure from Forward Head Tilt

To combat forward head posture and prevent nerve damage, she suggests, "Try performing shoulder blade squeezes and shrugging your shoulders up and down in a circular motion at your desk. These exercises remind the body to get out of the shrug and facilitate the mobility of muscles." These exercises are part of the Upper Body Rx described at the end of this chapter.

iPOSTURE HEADACHES

My clients with forward head posture often complain of frequent headaches. Many deskbound clients are surprised when they learn their stiff neck muscles are the cause. These are cervicogenic headaches, in which the pain from the cervical nerves in the C2 and C3 vertebrae radiates to the head and face. Dizziness and lightheadedness are also common symptoms of headaches from iPosture.

Heather, a forty-nine-year-old chief editor of a newspaper, was experiencing constant unilateral headaches on her right side for three years. She went to several doctors in search of a solution. Doctors thought she had migraines, but the migraine medication didn't help.

In the spring of 2019, a friend suggested that she see a chiropractor. The chiropractor diagnosed Heather with an excessively forward head position and linked her headaches to the muscle imbalance created by her iPosture. Then her chiropractor referred Heather to me.

After evaluation, I found that Heather's headaches were due to reduced stability. Her instability stemmed from the muscle imbalance around her neck and shoulder joints. The increased neck bend from tilting forward had tightened her chest muscles and weakened the muscles in her upper back. Also, her deep neck muscles in the front were weak, and the muscles at the back of her neck were tight.

iPosture Muscle Imbalances

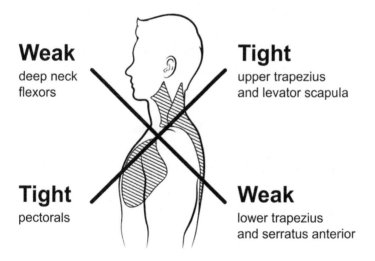

Weak
deep neck
flexors

Tight
upper trapezius
and levator scapula

Tight
pectorals

Weak
lower trapezius
and serratus anterior

Caption: iPosture Muscle Imbalance

I helped Heather with her iPosture muscle imbalance using corrective exercises to counteract the lack of equilibrium. Additionally, Heather bought a stand for her laptop to elevate the screen to eye level. You can find my laptop stand suggestion in the resources section. With eight weeks of a biweekly corrective exercise program, Heather's headaches decreased in intensity and frequency. Her new daily work routine now includes corrective exercises, breathing practice, and proper computer setup. Like Heather's headaches, there are many unusual symptoms we might not associate with poor posture.

Another notable symptom in my clients is pain behind the eyes, often accompanied by headaches. When it comes to eye strain, we don't naturally think of our posture. If we look closely at the internal workings of our upper body anatomy, it's easy to see all the major structures that control our vision lie in this region. The optic nerves pass through our cervical region. This nerve transmits electrical signals from the retina to the brain. Muscle tension in the upper back and neck can lead to eye strain and vision problems.

THE HUMPBACK

You might already be familiar with this postural dysfunction. Maybe your Aunt Doris had it in her later years. A client of mine, Brian, told me, "My mother is eighty years old and has a nasty hump. I'm concerned I'll have a hump just like my mother when I'm older."

At forty-five years old, he was already beginning to show signs of a kyphotic spine and was concerned about his posture because his mother had experienced spinal fractures. I worked on his kyphotic stance for twelve weeks, and his posture improved tremendously. His shoulder felt light after going through the corrective exercise program. I told Brian I was glad he got after the hump as soon as possible because our spine can be remolded with exercise and posture care if degeneration hasn't yet started.

A kyphotic spine sends pressure down the torso, leading to postural modifications at every joint. These adaptations decrease the stability needed to perform daily activities like walking on uneven surfaces, putting objects on an overhead shelf, and climbing stairs. It prompts an increased risk of falls and musculoskeletal injury and is also responsible for an increased mortality rate.

Productivity Tip: Tight chest muscles and a rounded upper back inhibit positive thinking, leading to less focus and productivity. To increase productivity, try stretching your chest by extending your arms in a wide T position out to the side, palms facing forward.

SHOULDER STRESS

When Tyler tried to open the refrigerator to get the creamer, he couldn't even reach for the handle because of throbbing pain in his right shoulder. He tried to elevate his arm overhead but was unable.

For the last six years, Tyler has worked as a financial analyst. The prior weekend he had been busy painting the nursery. When he sought help after the fridge incident, Tyler's doctor told him he had torn a rotator cuff because of his rounded shoulder posture. Painting the nursery put extra strain on his already stressed shoulder joint. On the doctor's recommendation, he completed eight weeks of physical therapy. After physical therapy, the pain was better, but after a long day at work, it would return. He came to see me to maintain his corrective exercise program.

I prescribed exercises for strengthening his rotator cuff and upper back muscles. Tyler found total pain relief in four months. He continues to practice corrective exercises regularly and takes postural breaks throughout the workday.

We can stop injuries like Tyler's by paying attention to our posture throughout the day, making simple changes in our workstation setup, and practicing corrective exercises.

COMPUTER SETUP FOR UPPER BODY

An optimal workstation setup that can help you to have a good posture is a great place to start:

- Place the monitor directly in front, so you don't have to turn your neck to look at it. For a dual-screen setup, strive for both screens to be in front instead of to the side.

- Placing the monitor about twenty-four inches from the head, about arm's length away, is a safe distance. Make sure the space is comfortable for your screen size.

- The top of the monitor should be at your eye level or slightly lower. Ergonomist Dr. Alan Hedge suggests, "When you are seated comfortably, a user's eyes should be in line with a point on the screen about 2–3 inches below the top of the monitor casing, not the screen" (Middlesworth 2015). You can use a laptop stand to help raise the screen height.

- Place the keyboard at the same height as your elbows. This will ensure your forearms are level and your wrists are neutral. Movable keyboard trays are an excellent tool to bring your keyboard down to elbow height. Using a Bluetooth keyboard and mouse can help promote a more neutral hand and wrist posture, leading to less strain on our hands.

I've included the suggestions in the resources at the end of this book. You can download these resources at www.aesha-tahir.com/books.

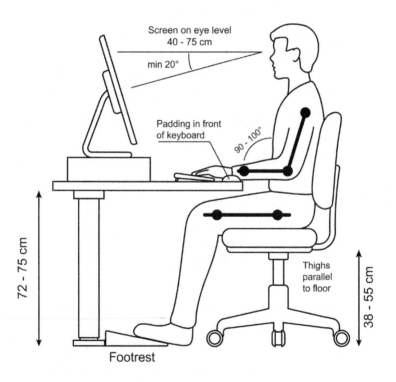

Caption: Proper Computer Setup

THE SECRET IS IN YOUR EYES

Your eyes are important postural system receptors. They help you orient your body in your environment. When you lift your arm in front, you know its position because the receptors in the eye define your sense of the arm's position. Monitor placement becomes crucial for our posture because it impacts the muscle imbalance of our eyes. Annette Verpillot, a posturologist, has worked extensively on how our posture is affected by the eyes and brain. She says on the TED stage, "Our posture is developed over time through our experience of the environment with our feet and our eyes" (TEDx Talks 2018).

Your eyes work in conjunction with your feet to orient your body in space. If the muscles of the eyes that move it side to side are imbalanced, that changes the proprioception of our environment and leads to compensation through our upper body muscles. Annette Verpillot detects and treats eye convergence disorders by correcting eye muscle imbalances. She suggests the following exercise to correct posture disorders due to eye imbalances.

- Draw a straight line about an inch long on the index finger of your dominant hand.

- Bring the index finger close to your body's midline and place it ten centimeters away from the root of the nose.

- Move your finger in a clockwise direction in front of your forehead, no higher than midforehead and no lower than midnose.

- Let your eyes focus on the drawn line and move clockwise with the finger.

- Perform this exercise for thirty seconds about three times a day.

The dominant index finger reconfigures the visual field like a magnet reconfigures the magnetic field. This exercise reeducates symmetrical movements between the right and left eye.

UPPER BODY RX

Simple stretching and strengthening exercises can restore our body's natural posture. These exercises counteract muscle imbalances and repetitive motion strain from sitting and typing. Working out at the gym is excellent, but this upper body exercise prescription is for anyone who works on a computer for long hours, regardless of their daily workout status.

ROLL AND RELEASE
Upper Back Release:

1. Lie with your back on a yoga mat or towel.

2. Place the foam roller horizontally under your upper back, close to your scapulae. Lift your hips slightly off the floor.

3. Roll back and forth over your upper back until you find a tight spot.

4. Hold the pressure at the tight spot for ninety seconds.

5. Move onto the next tight spot and repeat until the stiffness in your back is gone.

Posterior Shoulder Release:

For this exercise and the next, you can use a lacrosse ball for firm pressure or a tennis ball for soft pressure.

1. Lie with your back down on the yoga mat and your knees bent.

2. Place the massage ball behind your shoulder, connecting to the back muscles.

3. Gently rock back and forth in a circular motion until you find the tight spot.

4. Hold the pressure for ninety seconds at the tight spot.

5. Move onto the next sore spot and hold until your shoulder feels mobile.

Rhomboids Release:

1. Lie with your back on the floor or stand with your back against a wall.

2. Place the ball in the space between the spine and your shoulder blade.

3. Move the ball gently, rolling up and down until you feel a tender spot.

4. Hold on tender area for ninety seconds and remember to breathe.

STRETCHING EXERCISES
Chin Retraction:

1. Stand against a wall with your feet hip-distance apart, or if you have a chair with a backrest, you can stay seated.

2. Tuck your chin slightly down with two fingers and push your head back until it meets the wall or backrest.

3. Hold for five seconds before resting, and repeat five times.

4. Slowly build up to ten repetitions.

Neck Stretch:

1. While seated or standing at the desk, look up and over your shoulder.

2. Hold this position for ten seconds.

3. Repeat on the other side.

4. Perform three repetitions on each side.

Upper Back Stretch:

1. Place one hand on the side of your head and gently tilt it toward the shoulder on the same side.

2. Line your ears up with your shoulders like a chin tuck.

3. Press your head down until you can feel a good stretch going down the back of your neck.

4. Place your other hand behind your back.

Bruegger's Stretch:

1. Sitting in your chair, place your feet hip-distance apart.

2. Open your hands up and rotate your thumbs backward while extending your arms by your hips.

3. Relax your shoulders and let your shoulder blades slide down into your pants pockets.

4. Hold for twenty seconds and take deep breaths.

5. Repeat three to four times.

Bruegger's Stretch

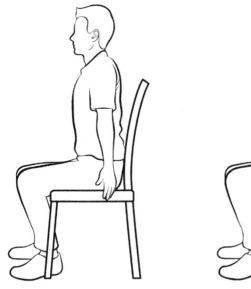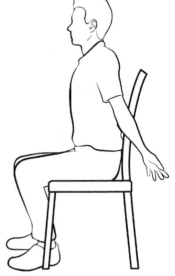

Caption: Seated Bruegger's Stretch

Standing Chest Stretch:

1. Stand in the corner of a room or to the side of the doorway.

2. Place your forearm against the wall with your elbow bent below shoulder level.

3. Push your torso forward until you feel a stretch in your chest muscles on the same side under your collarbone.

4. Hold for thirty seconds and practice on the second side.

5. Repeat after ten seconds of rest.

Seated Chest Stretch:

1. Sit in a comfortable position on your chair with your feet flat.

2. Spread your arms in a wide T position out to the side, palms facing forward. Think of the *Titanic* pose.

3. Extend your arms slightly behind your back until you feel the stretch in the front of your body around your shoulders and chest.

4. Hold the stretch for ten to twenty seconds.

5. Repeat four to five times during the day.

STRENGTH EXERCISES
Neck Extension:

1. Lie facedown on a yoga mat with your elbows stacked under your shoulders and forearms resting on the mat.

2. Lift your head off the mat and stretch it as far back as your body allows.

3. Feel the weight of your head strengthen your neck muscles.

4. Hold for twenty seconds and repeat three or four times.

Seated Shoulder Squeeze:

1. Relax your head, neck, and shoulders.

2. Bend your elbows, drawing your upper arms close to your chest and ribs.

3. Let your forearms come out to the side, almost parallel to the floor.

4. Squeeze the shoulders back and hold for ten seconds.

5. Release and repeat eight to ten times.

Desk Shoulder Rotation:

1. Pass a light or medium resistance band around one leg of your desk.

2. The resistance band should be at waist level. Tying the band around a doorknob is a good option if a desk's leg doesn't work.

3. Hold onto both ends of the resistance band while in a seated or standing position.

4. You can also hold a filled water bottle instead of a resistance band.

5. Rotate your hand away from your body while keeping the shoulder still.

6. Perform eight to ten repetitions.

Desk Rows:

1. Secure a resistance band around the front leg of your desk or a doorknob.

2. Grab one end of the band in each hand with your arms extended in front of you.

3. You can also use two water bottles instead of a resistance band.

4. Keep a slight bend in your elbows, with your wrists neutral.

5. Slowly pull the band back until your wrists are next to your waist.

6. Squeeze the shoulder blades together while pulling the band.

7. Hold the squeeze for three to four seconds.

8. Perform eight to ten repetitions.

Standing Ys:

1. Step on one end of the resistance band.

2. Hold the other end in the opposite hand or hold a water bottle in the other hand.

3. Slowly raise your hand with the band across your body as if forming the letter Y.

4. Stop at shoulder height.

5. Repeat eight to ten times.

Standing Scaptions:

1. Step on one end of a long resistance band.

2. Hold the other end in the opposite hand or hold a water bottle in the other hand.

3. Slowly raise your hand with the band in front of you at approximately a thirty-degree angle from your body, keeping your arm straight.

4. Stop at shoulder height.

5. Repeat eight to ten times.

UPSHOT OF iPOSTURE

The upshot of iPosture are the headaches, eye strain, shoulder injuries, and humpback. These conditions are our body's way of signaling pain from the distorted body posture we hold for long periods.

Posture Challenge: For a pain-free upper body, perform any three exercises from the Upper Body Rx plan daily. Our body can adapt to a better posture with practice, regular posture exercises, and movement breaks.

CHAPTER 13

At the Center of It

She returned to find her then-twenty-three-year-old husband lying on the floor in pain. She started scrambling frantically through her purse, hands trembling, looking for his pain medication and crying. After five long minutes, she finally found the medicine.

An hour after taking the pain medication, Angelo Poli got up and sat in his recliner with the help of his wife. Angelo was a strapping bodybuilder and a gym owner in Orland, California. He had injured his back while lifting weights a few months before this incident. After that, his health was on a slippery slope. He lost his balance often, and his lower back pain became so intense that he walked with a cane.

Over the next five years, he sought back pain relief through many methods. After trying many treatments, he found long-term relief when he met a coach who focused on posture and ergonomics. After that, he could stand straight and walk without a cane. After his experience, Angelo began incorporating posture correction with his own clients.

THE HIDDEN CAUSE OF BACK PAIN

Angelo Poli is known today for his work with elite athletes like the 2011 NFL MVP and World Record-holding powerlifters. "If you happen to be between eighteen and twenty-four years old, your odds of experiencing that back pain in the next twelve months increases," says Poli, standing on the red dot on stage (Poli 2013).

Our lower back is responsible for supporting the weight of our upper body. Persistently sinking into soft chairs increases the load on the lower back. Constant sitting induces an exaggerated curve in our spine, which reduces its ability to absorb shock. Poli explains, "When our body is under load in a biomechanically compromised position, we're going to suffer an injury. That injury can be sudden, and it can be catastrophic."

Muscles surrounding the spine protect us from such injuries. These muscles are fundamental for a healthy back. They carry the weight of our upper and lower body and act as an on-demand supportive brace when our body's load increases. The additional load can be functional, like with sports, exercise, and lifting your kids, or unhealthy, like unintentional weight gain. Ultimately, these muscles are responsible for every move we make.

WHAT IS THE CORE?

The core is quite the buzzword these days. Visit any fitness center or trainer's social media page, and you'll see core training is highlighted. Most people think the core is just the six-pack bodybuilders show off—but our core is much more expansive than that.

By definition, a core is the central or most important part of something. In our body, the core is the central region. It connects our upper body with the lower body, helping them operate in tandem. Muscles in our midsection, known as the lumbo-pelvic-hip complex, comprise the core. Thirty musculoskeletal structures are part of the core (Porterfield and DeRosa 1998).

There are three main groups of core muscles:

Deep Lumbar Spine Muscles: The muscles located deep inside our midsection drive our spinal movements. The psoas is the most notorious one and attaches to the pelvic bone right above the thigh in the front. The psoas is a deep hip flexor. You are probably familiar with this notorious muscle if you've suffered back pain. For deskbound professionals, the psoas is very tight and takes over the work of weak abdominal muscles. Prolonged sitting keeps our hips flexed and the psoas working even after hours when we are not sitting. It takes more than just standing up to let it relax.

Pelvic Muscles: The pelvic muscles, or glutes, are also part of the core. The significant pelvic floor muscles that affect our upright posture are the gluteus maximus, gluteus medius, and adductor muscles.

Abdominal Muscles: And last but not least, the iconic six-pack muscle is indeed part of this muscle group. The group it is a part of consists mainly of the superficially visible abdominal muscles in the front and side of our torso. Beneath the six-pack lies the external and internal oblique muscles. The deepest core muscle is the transverse abdominis, which wraps around our body like a corset. The transverse abdominis activates before the movement of arms and legs and compresses the abdomen while breathing.

The human spine depends upon activating all these muscles to provide stability. If stripped of these muscles, our spine would collapse under a meager twenty pounds of weight (Barr, Griggs, and Cadby 2005)

Think of our core as a soda can. When the can is unopened and filled with liquid, it's stable because of the pressure of the can's inner contents, so it will be hard to crush it by stepping on top. However, an empty soda can is much easier to stomp flat. Similarly, when our core muscles are engaged, they stabilize our spine to stay upright. But if these muscles are weak and inactive, it's easy to crush the core and compress our posture.

The most common reason for lower back pain is bending over or sitting with unengaged core muscles. Many of us sit in the same position for long stretches of time, causing our glutes and stabilizing core muscles to not fire properly. Instead, psoas and hamstrings compensate for the core inactivity.

THE ULTIMATE LINK IN YOUR BODY

Many clients ask me, "What is the one thing I can do to improve my posture?" My answer is always strengthening the core. It is the single best thing we can do to improve our posture.

I learned the importance of these muscles years back during physical therapy for my lower back pain. Through this healing process, I realized my psoas muscle was tight and my deep core muscles were weak. My core muscles weren't firing to support my movements and daily activities.

Above the core, you'll find structures such as the upper back and neck muscles. Knees, ankles, and systems that support them lie below the core. The forces produced by the lower body are transferred through the core to the upper body and vice versa. Pain-free and effective movements require core muscles to be strong.

Weak core muscles impair arm and leg functionality. Amy Selinger, a physical therapist specializing in back, hip, and pelvic pain at the Back to Life physical therapy practice in San Francisco, explained to me the importance of core muscles in an interview, saying, "Hodges and Richardson, two scientists, studied people with back pain and those without. They asked people to move their arms or to move their legs. They found that people without back pain turned on their abdominal muscles before anything happened in the arm or the leg. The other group with back pain couldn't turn on their abdominal muscles."

When you raise your hand to ask a question, your core muscles fire up first and stabilize your body for movement. But raising your hand will require other muscles to stabilize if your core muscles aren't strong, resulting in shoulder muscle fatigue and soreness. Amy outlines that "the abdominal muscles rush to catch up, so then the whole shack falls over because the periphery is stronger than the core."

Even a small amount of core weakness affects the whole kinetic chain. As with the spare tire on a car, we can't put many miles on it before it gives out.

MUSCLE WEAKNESS AND COMPENSATIONS

"If you sit a lot, odds are your buttock muscles are long, and your hip flexor muscles are short. Short muscles act strong, and long muscles act weak," Amy tells me, describing how our bodies compensate. "I see and treat a lot of people who have lower back pain, sacroiliac joint dysfunction, hip pain, painful intercourse, painful urination, or defecation because of this muscle imbalance."

CORE IMBALANCES

She also emphasized sitting in chairs for most of our lives primes us for a weak core. As a movement specialist, I agree with Amy's analysis. The BRACE model in this book addresses the muscular imbalances of the core complex that causes painful movement. Looking at the body as a whole unit that functions seamlessly from head to toe requires special attention toward core muscles.

When creating a corrective exercise program for my clients, the core is always at the center of it. I give gentle stretches for the tight muscles and strengthening exercises for the weak ones. I build a customized program for each client based on their postural dysfunctions. The three most common dysfunctions of the core complex are the anterior pelvic tilt, posterior pelvic tilt, and lateral tilt.

FORWARD TILT

Nathan, a marketing specialist for a pharmaceutical company, came to see me for lower back pain. At the initial consultation, I found that Nathan's pelvis tipped forward to keep his back straight. This muscular imbalance is called an anterior pelvic tilt, noticeable as an overly forward-arched lower back. Nathan having to sit for work caused his hip flexors to tighten because they were always bent. The tight muscles pulled his lower back forward, causing it to overextend (Starrett 2016). The opposing forces to the hip flexors, the abdominals, and the gluteus maximus, had become weak and lengthened, causing him pain. Over the next three months, we worked on strengthening Nathan's weak abs and glutes and stretching his psoas.

THE SECRET IS IN YOUR EYES

Your gaze impacts your body's position by stimulating your muscles to move in that direction. Our pelvis shifts forward when we look down at our computer screens because our brain treats it as an anticipatory movement signal in a forward direction and attempts to balance our center of gravity. This tilt results in an excessive lower back arch and pain. This reflex is called the pelvo-ocular reflex.

To keep the pelvo-ocular reflex in check, try these tips:

- Move your monitor screen arm's length away from your eyes and in direct line of sight.

- Be aware of the position of your head while working. Avoid bending it too far forward.

- Practice the 20-20-20 exercise. Every twenty minutes you spend on the screen, try to look at something straight twenty feet away for twenty seconds. It takes twenty seconds for your eye muscles to relax fully.

- Look straight ahead at the horizon while walking, hiking, and biking outdoors.

BACKWARD TILT

Another common postural deformity of weak core musculature is the posterior pelvic or hip tilt. People with hip tilt have a straight back with pelvic bones unnaturally tucked under the ribs. This positioning puts an extreme amount of pressure on the muscles supporting our spine. The glutes and low back muscles become weak, and abdominal muscles become tight, pulling the pelvis up (Takaki et al., 2016). This hip tilt causes back, joint, knee, and hip pain.

Laura has been battling back pain for years. When we met for a consultation, she told me, "I was a healthy high school and collegiate lacrosse player who never had any aches." But once she started medical school, her lifestyle changed dramatically: "I had to sit in the classroom studying for long hours. Then a few years later, during medical residency, I was on call at night, hunched over patients putting in IVs and doing lumbar punctures. That's when the back pain started." She went to see doctors, but after a while, she gave up on the regular epidural treatments, which were like putting a Band-Aid on her actual issue.

After an eight-week treatment program for a posterior pelvic tilt with her physical therapist, she continued her corrective exercise program with me. She has since seen a noticeable improvement in her back pain. Although she has some way to go, she is on the right track to addressing the real cause of her back pain.

LATERAL TILT

Much like being left- or right-handed, most of us have a preferred side of the body that we lean into. Try to notice which arm you use to brush your teeth or to reach for your clothes. This preference can have an impact on our spinal integrity. Our favoring of one side of the body creates a postural deformity called a lateral pelvic tilt. The quadratus lumborum, a muscle in the deep abdominal wall, is responsible for this postural distortion. When this muscle gets tight due to overuse on one side, it pulls the pelvis up on the opposite side (Al-Eisa, Egan, and Fenety 2004). The thigh, back of the leg, and outer leg muscles become tight on the side of the tilt.

Posture Tip: Don't sit on your wallet or phone. Many of my clients with a lateral pelvic tilt sit with an item in one of their back pockets. They unknowingly create a muscle imbalance. Even something as thin as a wallet keeps our pelvis from sitting level. It's best to take everything out of your back pockets before sitting.

We can address these postural dysfunctions by welcoming more movement into our daily routine. Attending a group exercise class that focuses on body alignments like Tai chi, yoga, and Pilates can also help core muscle strength. Regular corrective exercises for core muscles are another way to stay in the best posture.

TAKING CARE OF CORE AT THE DESK STATION

The key to protecting your lower back is to maintain the spine's normal curve. Supporting your back while working at your desk can help you do just that.

- Use a chair with a high-back, firm seat, and armrest. Sitting in a soft chair rounds the spine.

- Make sure your hips are attached to the back of the chair.

- If your chair doesn't have built-in back support, place a rolled towel between the curve of your spine and the back of your chair.

- Sit close to your desk so you don't have to reach and twist while working.

CORE RX

A consistent corrective exercise routine helps solve the core puzzle that eliminates lower back pain. Researchers in Korea studied the effect of core strengthening exercises (Ko et al. 2018). Participants in this study performed regular workouts three days a week for twelve weeks. The exercise regimen consisted of eight spinal stabilization exercises, part of my Core Rx program here. At the end of the study, participants reported decreased lower back pain and increased lumbar muscle strength and flexibility.

Try to incorporate the following core exercises into your daily routine.

ROLL AND RELEASE

Foam Roll Hip Flexors:

1. Lie face down with your forearms in front of you.

2. Place the lacrosse or tennis ball under your right hip.

3. Bend your left knee ninety degrees.

4. Roll up and down the front of your right hip bone.

5. If you find a tight spot, pause, and hold pressure on the region for ninety seconds.

6. Repeat the process on the next tight spot on this hip.

7. Repeat on your left hip.

Foam Roll Piriformis:

1. Place the foam roller under the back of your glutes.

2. Cross one leg over the other, placing your foot outside the opposite knee.

3. Slowly roll the back of the hip.

4. When you find a tight spot, pause for ninety seconds.

5. Repeat on your other side.

Foam Roll IT Band:

1. Lying on one side, place the foam roller under your hip perpendicular to the body.

2. Cross your top leg over your body, placing your foot on the floor.

3. Roll up and down along the outer thigh from the hip to the knee.

4. When you find a tight spot, pause for ninety seconds.

5. Repeat this process for the next tight spot on this side.

6. Repeat on the second side.

Foam Roll Low Back:

1. Lie on your back and press your feet firmly to the floor.

2. Hug your knees into your chest and place your hands on your shins.

3. Rock side to side.

4. Place the foam roller under your lower back for more intensity and follow the same steps.

5. Repeat three to four times.

STRETCHING EXERCISES

Seated Cats and Cows:

1. Sit tall on the front edge of your chair with your feet flat on the floor under your knees.

2. Place your hands on your thighs.

3. Inhale, arch your back, press your chest forward, and look up.

4. Exhale, round your neck and spine, and drop your chin to your chest.

5. Repeat six to eight times.

Chair Forward Fold:

1. Stand a few feet away from the back of the chair.

2. Slowly hinge forward at your hips until your hands lie on the chair.

3. Step back with your feet until your arms are straight.

4. Hold this stretch for ten to twenty seconds while taking deep breaths.

5. Let go of the back of the chair and then slowly roll up until you are standing up straight.

6. Repeat the chair fold three times.

Hip Flexor Stretch:

1. Step with your right foot forward and your left foot back.

2. Bend the front knee, stacking it on your ankle while keeping the back leg straight.

3. Place your hands on your desk for balance.

4. Hold for ten to twenty seconds, and then switch sides.

5. Repeat the chair fold three times on each side.

Seated Pigeon:

1. Sit tall in your chair with your back straight.

2. Place your right ankle on your left knee.

3. You should be able to feel a stretch in your right glute and outer thigh.

4. To intensify the stretch, hinge at your waist and drop your chest to your right lower leg.

5. Hold for ten to twenty seconds, then switch sides.

6. Repeat the seated pigeon three times on each side.

Seated Side Lunge:

1. While seated, extend your right leg to the right side and place your right heel on a footstool or an office box.

2. The left foot stays on the ground, stacked under the knee.

3. Slowly lean forward to intensify the inner thigh stretch.

4. Hold for ten to twenty seconds, then switch sides.

5. Repeat the seated side lunge three times on each side.

STRENGTH EXERCISES

Chair Sit-ups:

1. Sit straight in your office chair with your feet on the floor under your knees.

2. Place your hands on the side of the chair for support.

3. Keeping your lower back straight, move your chest toward your thighs.

4. Slowly lift your chest back up using your lower back muscles.

5. Optional: Place the resistance band under your feet if you are up for a bit more of a challenge. Hold each end of the resistance band in your hand and bend your chest closer to the thighs.

6. Perform eight to ten repetitions three to four times throughout the day.

Chair Twists:

1. Sit tall in a chair with your feet on the floor under your knees.

2. Extend your arms in front of your chest while holding a full water bottle.

3. Gently twist your body to the right, keeping your hips forward

4. Keep your hips attached to the chair and back long.

5. Hold the position for two seconds and then return to the starting position.

6. Repeat on the opposite side.

7. Perform eight to ten repetitions three to four times throughout the day.

Seated Boat:

1. Sit on your chair's front edge, pressing your legs together with your knees bent.

2. Lean back until your shoulders touch the backrest.

3. Hold the seat of your chair on either side.

4. While leaning back, slowly draw your knees in toward your chest.

5. Extend your legs out in front of you and hold for a second.

6. Keeping the legs lifted off the floor, pull the knees into your chest again.

7. Optional: You can keep one leg on the floor and pull one knee up into the chest at a time for better balance.

8. Perform eight to ten repetitions three to four times throughout the day.

Superman:

1. Lie on a yoga mat facedown, extending your arms in front of you.

2. Raise your arms and chest off the floor at the same time.

3. Hold the lifted chest for two seconds while exhaling.

4. Slowly lower your arms and chest back down while inhaling.

Dead Bugs:

1. Lie with your back flat on the yoga mat.

2. Extend your arms with a finger pointing up to the ceiling, in line with your shoulders.

3. Lift your legs into a tabletop position with your knees over your hips.

4. Engage your core by sinking your belly button toward your spine. Keep your lower back glued to the mat without any gap between them.

5. Move one arm behind you and lower the opposite leg toward the floor.

6. Bring the arm and leg back up to starting position.

7. Repeat on the opposite side.

8. Perform eight to ten repetitions three to four times throughout the day.

Hip Bridge:

1. Lie flat on the mat without any gap between the mat and your lower back.

2. Bend your knees, with your feet hip-distance apart and heels close to your hips.

3. Place your arms at the side and hands near your hips.

4. Lift the hips upward while squeezing your glutes and pushing your heels into the mat.

5. Create a straight line from your shoulders to your knees.

6. Hold for two seconds, then slowly lower back until your lower back is resting on the mat.

7. Perform eight to ten repetitions three to four times throughout the day.

UPSHOT OF A WEAK CORE

The upshot of the weak core complex is that it leads to musculoskeletal issues, which travel up to our shoulders and down to our feet. It's like having a house with unstable foundations. Lower back pain and other musculoskeletal disorders often result from a suboptimal core complex strength. To prevent these issues and lead a healthier life, we must understand the proper functioning of the core and positioning of the pelvis. With a better understanding of musculoskeletal structures, implementing a consistent workout routine encompassing the appropriate corrective exercises will help lead to a pain-free back and body.

Posture Challenge: I invite you to incorporate some of these exercises into your daily routine.

CHAPTER 14

Walk This Way

———

Supermodels need a smooth one. Toddlers need a balanced one. Politicians need a confident one. Can you guess what it is?

It's the way they walk, also called their gait. From iconic runways to blockbuster movies, we've all seen someone with a gait that draws our attention.

What can others learn from your gait? You might want to ask a psychopath. Chillingly, psychopaths choose their victims by looking at how they walk. A 2013 study at a maximum-security prison showed that psychopathic murderers could accurately access a person's vulnerability 100 percent of the time by how they walked (Book, Costello, and Camilleri 2013). People can gauge emotional stability, adventurousness, extraversion, trustworthiness, and warmth by the swing or sway in a person's gait. It's a window into much more than your emotions.

Your gait is a biometric trait, just like your fingerprints. It involves every body part, from your brain's neurologic feedback to the smallest muscles of your foot. A person's footprint can tell us about their lower body health.

FOOT

Feet are your only connection with the ground. Because of this, the foot is often the first clue that there might be muscle dysfunction which could lead to pain and injury. If any part of the foot isn't functioning well, muscular adaptions will appear in the rest of your leg.

Together, both feet comprise 25 percent of the body's bones, 18 percent of joints, and 6 percent of the muscles (Dimon and Qualter 2008). Your foot connects to your body at the ankle joint with two bones: the tibia and fibula. These bones connect to the big thigh bone (the femur) at the knee joint. The femur's head inserts into the pelvis, completing the connection to core complex. How your foot strikes the ground can affect muscles throughout your body.

Our feet have to do a lot of work besides just holding our weight. While moving, your foot must adapt to the ground surface, aid in shock absorption, and act as a lever to propel the body forward. Proper foot side-to-side motion is critical to achieving optimal movement. This side-to-side weight shift in the foot can also occur when we stand up, but the effects compound in a dynamic environment. Dr. Suresh Sivacolundhu, a podiatrist at The Foot Clinic in Perth, Australia, says, "Pronation is a very normal movement. What we get to see here is either excessive pronation or not enough pronation or some sort of abnormal pronation" (Sivacolundhu 2018).

OVERPRONATION

Twenty-one percent of the world's adult population have overpronated foot posture (Sánchez-Rodríguez et al. 2012). The increased inward roll of our foot and the arch collapse causes the leg to turn inward, affecting the knees, hips, and lower back posture. In a YouTube video, Dr. Paul Johnson, a podiatrist at the Yorkshire Sports Podiatry and Gait Clinic, says, "After the heel lands, the ankle rolls way to the inside. This forces the big toe to do most of the work needed to push off the ground again" (Johnson n.d.).

When this occurs, the inner lower leg muscles become overactive, and the anterior outer leg muscles weaken. The calf muscles in the back of the leg also become tight. This misalignment of the joints causes the foot to become structurally weak. The muscles, tendons, and ligaments of the lower leg work harder to stabilize the foot, possibly leading to injuries. Even two to three degrees of increased foot pronation leads to a 50–75 percent greater lower back arch during walking. An overly arched lower back can result in lower back pain or even spinal injuries and might lead to soft tissue injuries like muscle and ligament tears at the knee and hip joints.

SUPINATION

Just like our arch collapses too far inward while overpronating, it can also collapse outward. This outward collapse is called supination. To explain, Dr. Johnson says, "The heel strikes first, the weight transfers to the outside of the foot, and it stays there, so [we push] off the outer toes to begin the next stride." This type of outward foot movement is common among people with high arches. It causes the external rotation of our legs and places extra stress on the outer leg muscles, creating a muscle imbalance in the lower leg. "It puts added pressure on your lower legs that can lead to injuries," Dr. Johnson cautions. Supinators experience pain in joints, ankle sprains, calluses, or bunions on the outer edge of the foot, and inflammation of the outer thigh and hip muscles.

Both foot muscle irregularities cause most of our weight to transfer to the outer edges of our foot, but overpronation is nine times more common than supination. This is because of excessive sitting during the workday: Long periods of sitting weaken our gluteal muscles, which allow the collapsing of the medial arch of the foot and, in many cases, lead to flat feet.

Megan had been experiencing heel pain on the inner edge of her feet for about eight months before she came for treatment in November 2019. The pain was worst first thing in the morning when she woke up. She worked from home as a data analyst and had recently adopted a dog to be active, but her heel pain was discouraging, and she couldn't walk the dog that often. During her standing posture and gait analysis, she rolled her feet inward.

Megan had plantar fasciitis. The plantar fascia is a layer of connective tissue spanning under the foot from the toes to the heel. This condition is prevalent in deskbound professionals because of their sedentary lifestyle. Upon further analysis, her calf muscles were tight, and her glutes were weak. She started feeling better after implementing a corrective exercise program for eight weeks. Exercise is the best intervention for correcting musculoskeletal disorders created by improper posture. These exercises are part of the Lower

Body Rx program mentioned below. You can watch plantar fascia care videos at www.aeshatahir.com/books.

TAKING CARE OF LEGS AT THE DESK STATION

Proper foot posture is vital to keep your body correctly aligned. Some interventions to improve weight distribution in your feet while sitting or standing at your desk are:

- While seated at your desk station, push your hips as far back as possible in the chair.

- Adjust the chair height so your feet are flat on the floor and your knees are equal to, or slightly lower than, your hips. When knees are higher than hips, pressure increases on the knees.

- If your chair isn't adjustable, place your feet flat on a foot-stool or box.

- Wear flexible and lightweight shoes. Avoid high heels, flats, and flip-flops while working. The best way to find a comfortable shoe is to go to an athletic or medical shoe shop and get fitted for a comfortable pair. If you like to work barefoot, investing in a good, cushioned foot mat under your desk will help.

- If you have been diagnosed with overpronation or supination, insoles designed for these postural dysfunctions can support the arch and heel to control foot movement. You can buy these insoles online or at your local shoe store.

- When you walk, try to land softly on the feet from heel to toe. A short stride is best to ensure proper walking form. Incorporating walking breaks throughout the day is essential to loosen tight muscles and strengthen weak foot muscles.

KNEES

The most common ailment I see is pain in the knees. Knee pain is the second most chronic musculoskeletal condition globally, falling just behind lower back pain (Uyen-Sa D T et al. 2011). In fact, frequent knee pain limits the functioning and mobility of 25 percent of adults. Posture distortions at the ankle and hip joints transfer the sheer forces to the knee joint, resulting in pain.

This joint is supported by a network of muscles, and a muscle imbalance around the knee joint causes the knee to become unstable. The instability of the knee joint can be linked to two significant postural imbalances: knocked knees and bowed knees.

KNOCKED KNEES

The knocked knee is characterized by the inward bend of the knees, where thigh bones rotate inward and the feet turn inward.

Next time you stand or sit, notice if your knees are pointing forward or crossing your big toe and pointing inward. Accompanying knocked knees are flat feet or a collapsed arch like the overpronated foot posture. Knocked knees can be genetic, but we will explore the condition in relation to poor posture in this book.

Two renowned physical therapists, Dr. Bob Schrupp and Dr. Brad Heinicke, think one cause can be "the footwear, tight muscles, [and] some of the activities [people] do" (Schrupp and Heineck 2016). In the YouTube video discussing this, Dr. Schrupp points to the inner thigh, saying, "When these muscles are tight, they pull the knee inward, which helps to knock [them toward the midline of the body]." In people with knocked knees, the inner thigh muscles are tight, and the outer thigh muscles are weak.

Knocked knees can lead to arthritis in the outer part of the knees because knocked knee posture compresses the ligaments on the outer side. Pointing to the inside of the knee on the skeleton model, Dr. Schrupp says, "You have a gap here between these bones at this side of the joint, which means it is not going to wear out at all on this side."

Then he explains when the outside of the knee and ligament get compressed, "You have much more risk of developing arthritis in the lateral compartment or the outside of the knee." If left untreated, knocked knees can progress and cause symptoms like limping, osteoarthritis, lower back pain, and ankle pain.

BOWED KNEES

Some postural imbalances can cause the knees to fan outward. When the muscles on the outside of the knee become dominant, the result is bowed knees. Imagine the knees forming a diamond shape while standing and walking: The person's legs bend outward, and their knees don't touch even when the feet are together.

This is because the outer thigh muscles pull the kneecap to the outside, and the inner thigh muscles become weak. The inner side of the knee joint compresses, and the thigh bone rubs against the lower leg bone. There are many causes of this distorted posture, from heredity to previous injury, but in my practice, it is common among clients who sit for prolonged periods and put their weight on the outside edges of their feet.

Kenneth, forty-eight, came to see me because of a dull month-long outer thigh pain after a short run in September 2019. For the last four years, he has been an avid walker and wellness champion at his financial investment company. Upon his posture evaluation, I noticed he put his weight on the pinky toe and outer edges of his feet while getting out of a chair. Then, in the standing position, his knee pointed outward.

Ken had bowed knees and supinated feet. This postural dysfunction led to IT band Syndrome, which causes a dull ache in the outer thigh. The iliotibial (IT) band is a thick band of fibrous tissue that runs outside the leg and can become inflamed when overused, which is what caused Ken's knee pain.

I worked with Ken to stretch his outer thigh muscles and strengthen his inner thigh and gluteus muscles. Evenly distributing his weight all over his foot and activating his big toe and ball of his foot while walking and standing was part of the posture protocol. Ken foam rolled his outer thigh regularly. He also performed seated inner thigh squeezes, bridges, and flat back leg extensions to strengthen his muscles. Both these exercises are part of the Lower Body Rx program below. After eight weeks, Ken's knee pain subsided.

Bowed knees can lead to degenerative changes on the inner edge of the knee and to arthritis and other soft tissue injuries. The good news is that bowed knees due to muscle imbalance can be corrected with exercise and postural awareness if caught early.

LOWER BODY RX

Again, exercise is the best way to treat postural dysfunctions. Corrective exercise improves the gait and reduces overpronation within six months. The exercises below can be implemented daily as a part of your posture break to realign the knee and ankle and reduce pressure on these joints.

ROLL AND RELEASE
Tennis Ball Rolls:

1. Stand with your feet flat on the floor.
2. Place a tennis ball or lacrosse ball under one foot.
3. Standing straight, roll the ball back and forth under the foot for two minutes.
4. Switch and repeat with the other foot.

Foam Roll Calf Muscles:

1. Sit on a yoga mat or a towel with your legs extended in front of you.

2. Place the roller horizontally under the lower leg.

3. Roll back and forth over the calf muscles while the toe points toward the sky.

4. Lift your glutes slightly off the mat by pushing your hands behind them.

5. Apply light to moderate pressure on tight spots.

6. Hold for sixty seconds, then move on to the next tight location.

7. Repeat these steps on the other leg.

Foam Roll Outer Thighs:

1. Lie on a yoga mat or towel on one side of your body.

2. Place the foam roller under the bottom hip.

3. Use the bottom arm to slowly roll down from hip to knee.

4. Apply light to moderate pressure on tight spots.

5. Hold for sixty seconds, then move on to the next tight spot.

6. Switch to the other side and repeat.

Foam Roll Inner Thighs:

1. Lie facedown with your forearms in front of you on the mat.

2. Lift your head, neck, and chest off the mat.

3. Bring one leg out to the side with your knee bent, so your inner thigh is perpendicular to the mat.

4. Place the foam roller under the inner thigh.

5. Use your arms to roll up and down along your inner thigh by moving side to side.

6. Hold medium pressure on tight spots for thirty to sixty seconds.

7. Repeat on the other side.

STRETCHING EXERCISES
Heel Stretch:

1. Stand with your feet hip-distance apart in front of a wall.

2. Step forward with one foot until your front toes touch the wall.

3. Bend the front knee and lean forward at your hips, transferring most of the weight to the front foot.

4. Keeping the spine long, press your hands into the wall while the back leg straightens.

5. Feel the stretch in the calf muscles of the back leg.

6. Hold for thirty seconds, then switch legs.

7. Repeat four times.

You can also do this exercise by holding the edge of a desk.

Seated Inner Thigh Stretch:

1. Sit on the floor and bring the soles of your feet together.

2. Move your feet toward your tailbone.

3. Hold onto your ankles and bend your chest forward until you feel a pull in your inner thigh muscles.

4. Keep your back straight and aligned as you bend at your hips.

Seated Outer Thigh Stretch:

1. Sit tall in your chair with your back attached to the back-rest and hips under your shoulders.

2. Plant your left foot on the floor.

3. Place your right ankle on your left thigh close to the knee. Your legs should form a figure four in this stretch.

4. Press your bent knee toward the floor.

5. Feel the stretch in the muscles of your outer hips and thigh.

6. Hold for thirty to sixty seconds and repeat on the second side.

STRENGTH EXERCISES

Calf Raises:

1. Stand behind your chair, holding onto the back of it.

2. Start with both feet on the ground and hip-distance apart.

3. Lift both heels as high as possible, hold for five seconds, then lower them.

4. Repeat ten to fifteen times.

Toe Raises:

1. Stand with both feet on the floor.

2. Press the right big toe into the floor and lift the other toes of the right foot.

3. Hold for five seconds.

4. Next, press the four smaller toes into the floor and raise the big toe for five seconds.

5. Repeat each exercise five to ten times.

6. Repeat with the other foot.

Inner Thigh Squeeze:

1. Sit upright in your chair with a toilet paper roll between your knees.

2. Clench your glutes and gently squeeze the toilet paper roll.

3. Hold the squeeze for five seconds.

4. Perform eight to ten repetitions.

Seated Hip Abduction:

1. Sit tall in your chair with your back straight and soft shoulders.

2. Tie or pull the resistance band on your thighs above your knees.

3. Place your feet hip-width apart with heels under your knees.

4. Push your knees away from each other as far as your body allows.

5. Slowly bring them back together.

6. Perform eight to ten repetitions.

UPSHOT OF LOWER BODY

Your feet bear the weight of your body. Proper foot posture that distributes the body weight evenly is essential for optimal movement and stability. Your knees are the center of your legs that help your body propel forward, and a muscle imbalance at the knee can distort your movement and lead to early degeneration of the joint. These lower extremity distortion patterns can lead to a chain reaction of muscle imbalances and structural problems that spread to the rest of your body.

Posture Challenge: Take short ten-minute breaks three or four times a day at work to release, stretch, and strengthen your lower leg muscles. These exercises can help you avoid muscle imbalances and chronic musculoskeletal diseases like arthritis.

Daily Workout Plan

As we've learned, postural health has four pillars: breath, relaxation, activity, and corrective exercise. The goal is to incorporate all four pillars into your daily routine. Over time, you will start thinking about the pillars as a holistic model that works together. I've put together a sample schedule that includes the four pillars you learned in this book. You can follow this workout plan or make your own. The ultimate goal is better posture.

	BREATH	RELAXATION	ACTIVITY	COR. EXERCISE
MONDAY	Morning: Diaphragmatic breathing Evening: Diaphragmatic breathing	Lunch: 3 Upper Body Stretches Lunch: Quiet Time*** 3-minutes	Lunch: Walk 10–20 minutes	Evening: Warmup* 10-minutes Evening: 3 Upper Body Strength Exercises
TUESDAY	Morning: Diaphragmatic breathing Lunch: Alternate nostril breathing	Lunch: 3 Core Stretches Lunch: Guided Meditation** 3–5 minutes	Morning: Walk 10–20 minutes	Evening: Warmup 10- minutes Evening: 3 Lower Body Strength Exercises
WEDNESDAY	Morning: Box breathing Evening: Diaphragmatic breathing	Lunch: 3 Lower Body Stretches Lunch: Guided Meditation 3-minutes	Lunch: Walk 10–20 minutes	Evening: Warmup 10- minutes Evening: 3 Upper Body Strength Exercises

Day				
THURSDAY	Morning: Diaphragmatic breathing Lunch: Alternate nostril breathing	Lunch: 3 Upper Body Stretches Lunch: Quiet Time 3-minutes	Morning: Walk 10–20 minutes	Evening: Warmup 10- minutes Evening: 3 Core and Lower Body Strength Exercises
FRIDAY	Morning: Diaphragmatic breathing Evening: Diaphragmatic breathing	Lunch: Upper Body Stretches Lunch: Guided Meditation 3–5 minutes	Lunch: Walk 10–20 minutes	Evening: Warmup 10-minutes Evening: 3 Upper Body Strength Exercises
SATURDAY	Morning: Diaphragmatic breathing Evening: Diaphragmatic breathing	Lunch: 3 Upper Body and 3 Core Stretches	Morning: Walk 10–20 minutes Lunch: Light Cardio	Evening: Warmup 10-minutes Evening: 3 Core and 3 Lower Body Strength Exercises
SUNDAY	Morning: Diaphragmatic breathing Lunch: Box breathing	Lunch: 3 Upper Body Stretches	Lunch: Walk 10–20 minutes	Evening: Warmup 10-minutes Evening: 3 Core and 3 Lower Body Stretches

*Warmup: Any light cardio or walk to get the blood circulating will improve the efficiency of your exercise.

**Guided Meditation: You can find guided meditations at www.aeshatahir.com/books

***Quiet Time: This is the white space during the day. Try to do nothing during this time by removing yourself from all sensory experiences.

Conclusion
Simple Solutions for Modern Humans

Small postural health habits led to significant changes for Karen. She started slowly with these habits and then consistently applied them. After six months of corrective exercise intervention, her headaches were relieved, and she could slowly get back to swimming. Her neck muscles have optimal strength, and now she swims regularly twice a week. Two years in, she lowered her LDL cholesterol (bad cholesterol) by ten points and lost twenty pounds. The higher metabolic rate was just a byproduct of her better postural habits. She has consistent energy throughout the day and has been very productive. She is an effective leader for her team at work and for her family at home. She truly feels emotionally empowered by this transition. She was promoted in July 2022 to Vice President of Technology due to her higher productivity.

Karen was the first client who inspired me to write about the postural issues affecting modern deskbound professionals.

This idea led to two years of data collection, pattern recognition, research, and many interviews. My interviews ranged from expert anthropologists for understanding human origins to pulmonologists for understanding how breathing is connected to posture. During this time, I've learned proper posture has tremendous benefits throughout our body, from eliminating musculoskeletal disorders to effective leadership, from pain-free movement to better mental health. The benefits of posture on our health became more evident as I put the pieces of my book's puzzle together.

The journey that started in December 2020, after Karen's consultation, has led me to many vital lessons on the importance of posture and how to preserve it—beginning with the effect of zero gravity on astronauts. The gravitational force provides the necessary resistance for our muscles and bones to stay upright and perform functional movements. Our upright skeletal structure today evolved due to the force of gravity on our quadrupedal ancestors' bodies. Louis the Gorilla reminded me of our common ancestors. We became unhunched because it provided a survival advantage for our species. But we are not done evolving. Our bodies are constantly changing and responding to environmental stress.

It makes me wonder where our species is headed with our current postural state and sedentary lifestyle. Evidence suggests overusing technology in a hunched stance leads to our species' dys-evolution. It can change our skeleton into a deformed shape with curled hands, hunched backs, and smaller brains. Anthropologists are doing fantastic research and work to understand the past so we can build a better future. I'm confident we will have many more answers on how we can preserve our postural health to help the survival of our species. Taking a leaf out of the lifestyle of today's indigenous populations might provide us with a better way to sit, stand and perform our daily activities.

The BRACE model gets to the root cause behind pain, anxiety, and metabolic diseases our species is experiencing. Suppose you are working hunched over your desk, unaware of your breathing, mental stress, activity level, and muscle imbalances. In that case, this book has all the tools for healing yourself by introducing small behavior changes that honor your evolutionary physiology.

Learning to sit, stand, and move with an aligned spine requires a balanced action from all muscle groups. Some muscles naturally take over the work due to their ability to fire quickly. Corrective exercises can help you to strengthen the muscles your body needs to fire when working and moving. These corrective exercise routines are a new tool in your wellness toolbox.

Creating wellness cultures at work would reinforce these behaviors. As I write this section of the book after presenting the "Stand Up for Posture" workshop to a group of entrepreneurs this morning, I realize how much people want to take control of their health. They want access to tools that prevent physical and emotional pain. They are willing to take responsibility for their health and take small steps to build a balanced, strong, powerful body and brain.

That's what this book is all about. It serves as a North Star for your natural posture. It might take some time to see the results, but consistency will help turn these better postural habits into automatic behavior. When you are learning how to drive, you need to make a conscious effort to control the car, but with time you can operate the vehicle without much effort because of the habits you've developed.

We need to create new connections in our brains to change an established habit and adopt a new behavior. The first step in behavior change is awareness. After reading this book, you have the understanding to develop postural changes. Small changes repeatedly over time build stronger brain connections, making the new healthier posture a habit. Small changes can be setting a timer to do stretching exercises from this book every thirty minutes, going for a ten-minute walk before starting your day, taking a movement lunch, practicing deep breathing daily for five minutes, or changing your working position every thirty minutes. These small changes compound and lead to better postural habits.

My hope from this book is that it gives you knowledge about better posture and a model to follow that will help you stay motivated and increase your resilience to overcome setbacks in the way of positive posture changes. You can improve your posture and live a pain-free and healthy life regardless of age.

All you need to do is start making small changes. The power is in your hands!

Resources

———

I've found many of my clients are looking for tools to support their posture. Below is a list of resources mentioned in the book. These are some suggestions. There are many brands out there making these products. Feel free to swap them with another brand of your choice.

Floor Desk: I like the Cooper Mega Floor Desk. This is a folding floor desk that folds to a height of 10.6 inches and features a 25.6″ × 19.3″ work area.

Desk Converter: I like the VIVO 32-inch Sit to Stand Desk Converter. It's an adjustable height desk converter with a keyboard stand. You can also use this as a floor desk.

Electric Standing Desk: I like FLEXISPOT EN1 Electric White Stand Up Desk with a lot of space and touch adjustable height buttons.

Ergo Chair: Any chair with a backrest and sturdy seat is good for posture. When you try the chair, make sure the seat has a cushion for comfort, but it's not so soft that you sink into it. I like the ERGOUP Ergonomic Office Chair

Laptop Stand: KENTEVIN Adjustable Laptop Stand raises the laptop screen.

Ergo Mouse and Keyboard: It's easy to place a portable Bluetooth mouse and keyboard close to you for better arm posture. I like the Kensington Pro Fit Ergo Wireless Keyboard and Mouse.

What's Next

———

Thank you for reading this book all the way through. It's a pleasure to share my experience and knowledge with amazing readers like you. If you liked this book, I'd like to suggest that you check out weekly articles on my website aeshatahir.com/articles. You can also check out weekly posture snacks on my YouTube channel, Tone and Strengthen. I think you'll like them.

If this book has helped you, it really helps me if you leave a review on Amazon or Goodreads. I personally read every posted review. I update the posture exercise library regularly to activate even more muscles and create muscle balance. Take a quick look now at www.aeshatahir.com/bookupdates. Finally, if you want to get in touch, my email is info@aeshatahir.com and you can add me on social media as @AeshaTahir on most platforms.

Acknowledgments

——

I felt elated as I finished writing this book. Writing a book is more challenging than I thought and more rewarding than I could have ever imagined. My early drafts were a mess, and the revision process was grueling. There were many sleepless nights. If you know me, that was a big undertaking. There were missed workouts, sprained ankles, lost weekends, Door-Dash deliveries for kids, and many missed social events. This journey is comparable to my athletic endeavors. Like running a marathon, the buildup was challenging, and the last few miles were the most difficult. As I typed the final words, I felt the endorphins of crossing the finish line.

I relied heavily on many cheerleaders throughout this race. I want to start by thanking my incredible husband, Farhan, without whose encouragement I wouldn't have embarked on this journey. He played many roles during the writing process: spouse, friend, critic, kids' Uber driver, and chief marketing officer. He was as important to this book getting done as I was. Thanks to my kids, Rayan, Aydin, and Nyle, for their patience and for giving me the time to create and finish this book.

I'm grateful to my family for believing in me. For the encouragement and support I received from my dad and mom. I want to thank my sister Amber for her listening ear and the therapy sessions throughout the book writing process.

Thanks to my leadership coaches, Deborah Linett and Val Hastings, for helping me reach my potential and achieve this dream. Special thanks to my speech coach Jessica Iglesias for being my sounding board and listening to me read every draft of this book.

As for the content of this book, I have a long list of people to thank. Many people helped me figure out many of the fine details. I'm immensely thankful to Laura Templeton, Debbie Bellenger, Nithya Bhatt, Ritesh Bhatt, Ayoade Lawrence, Raghusai Kuntamukkala, Ana Malovrh, Tonia Tyler, Brandy Hollaway, Christina Smith, and Zuri Star for honest conversations and shaping the message of this book. Thanks to Dr. Kyle Stull for helping me figure out the nuances of the concept. To Prof. Eric Koester for offering me the perfect vehicle to channel my experience. Thanks to my illustrator Shawn Lin for creating phenomenal graphics for this book. To the team at Manuscripts who made this book a reality. Special thanks to the editors and marketing specialists for their guidance at every step of the publishing process.

Thanks to those who took time out of their busy schedules to read the early drafts of the manuscript, including Ayoade Lawrence, Deborah Linett, Neetu Shah, Nirav Shah, Maureen Benoit, and David Young. The book benefitted greatly from your feedback.

Thanks to all the supporters of my presale campaign, including Dolores Torsitano, Nithya Bhatt, Raghusai Kuntamukkala, Susan Mellinger, Gwynne Bee, Jody Rook, Kristy Crippen, Ayoade Lawrence, Ambreen Rana, Linda Alfino, Maureen Benoit, Paula Gasper, Faizah Zuberi, David Young, Debbie Bellenger, Megha Reddy, Jalal Shawwa, Melissa Merkle, Shayma Kazmi, Judith Ring, Deborah Linett, Kenneth Bingener, Faith Schlegel, Neetu Dhawan, Carolyn Johnson, Tom Schultz, Faith McManimon, Aarti Gupta, Caleb Ing, Jennifer Stoltz, Laura Templeton, Lise McFarlane, Stacy Ravindranathan, Deepa Mukund, Martha Williams, Sabahath Jaleel, Mona Soomro, Ana Malovrh, Mark Boyer, Melissa Jester, Nelson Scott, and Eric Koester.

Every author faces obstacles and low moments when writing. There were many people who offered me kind words of encouragement to carry on. Thanks to Dr. James Smith Jr. for his heartening phone call. Thanks to my running coach Charlotte Gould for helping me cross yet another finish line with supportive words.

Finally, thanks to you for taking the time to read this book and sharing it with others. I know if enough of us learn about posture, we can lead healthy and empowered lives.

My heart fills with all the love and support I've received in life. I will never be able to acknowledge all the beautiful people who have made the dream of writing this book a reality.

Appendix

———

INTRODUCTION: CAVEPERSON'S WELLNESS GUIDE

AANS. 2009. "Scoliosis—Symptoms, Diagnosis and Treatment." https://www.aans.org/Patients/Neurosurgical-Conditions-and-Treatments/Scoliosis.

APA. 2006. "Multitasking: Switching Costs." https://www.apa.org, March 20, 2006. https://www.apa.org/topics/research/multitasking.

American Chiropractic Association. 2020. "Back Pain Facts and Statistics." ACA Hands Down Better, May 19, 2020. https://handsdownbetter.org/health-and-wellness/back-pain-facts-and-statistics/.

Guardian Staff Reporter. 2018. "Usain Bolt Breaks World Record in Time of 9.58sec to Win 100m Gold in Berlin." *The Guardian*, February 21, 2018. https://www.theguardian.com/sport/2009/aug/16/usain-bolt-world-record-100m-world-athletics-championships.

Health Policy Institute. 2019. "Chronic Back Pain." Health Policy Institute, February 13, 2019. https://hpi.georgetown. edu/backpain/.

Howard, Desmond. 2011. Review of Bolt: "I Want to Do Wild Things." ESPN, November 29, 2011. https://www.espn.com/ olympics/story/_/id/7294360/olympics-usain-bolt-being-fastest-man-world-espn-magazine.

Hazlegreaves, Steph. 2019. "Office Workers Spend 75% of Their Waking Hours Sitting Down." Open Access Government. August 14, 2019. https://www.openaccessgovernment.org/ office-workers-sitting-down/71612.

World Health Organization. 2022. "Indicator Metadata Registry Details." https://www.who.int/data/gho/indicator-metadata-registry/imr-details/3416.

CHAPTER 1: PULL OF POSTURE

Bettany-Saltikov, J., and L. Cole. 2012. "The Effect of Frontpacks, Shoulder Bags and Handheld Bags on 3D Back Shape and Posture in Young University Students: An ISIS2 Study." *Studies in Health Technology and Informatics* 176: 117–21. https://pubmed.ncbi.nlm.nih.gov/22744472.

Clément, Gilles. 2005. *Fundamentals of Space Medicine.* Dordrecht: Springer Netherlands.

Flinn, Allie. 2019. "This Is the Absolute Worst Bag for Your Posture, According to a Chiropractor." Well+Good.

September 11, 2019. https://www.wellandgood.com/worst-bag-for-posture/.

Kendall, Florence P., et al. 2010. *Muscles: Testing and Function with Posture and Pain.* Baltimore, MD: Lippincott Williams & Wilkins.

Seibert, Günther. 2001. *Bulletin Agence Spatiale Européenne.* European Space Agency.

Shackelford, Linda C. 2008. "Musculoskeletal Response to Space Flight." *Principles of Clinical Medicine for Space Flight,* 293–306. https://doi.org/10.1007/978-0-387-68164-1_14.

CHAPTER 2: BECOMING UNHUNCHED

Choi, Charles Q. 2017. "Fossil Reveals What Last Common Ancestor of Humans and Apes Looked Like." *Scientific American,* August 10, 2017. https://www.scientificamerican.com/article/fossil-reveals-what-last-common-ancestor-of-humans-and-apes-looked-liked/.

Desmond, Adrian. 2023. "Charles Darwin | Biography, Education, Books, Theory of Evolution, & Facts." *Encyclopedia Britannica,* January 5, 2023. https://www.britannica.com/biography/Charles-Darwin.

Fox, Daniel. 2018. "At Philly Zoo, Louis the Gorilla Takes Great Strides to Round up Snacks." WHYY. March 29, 2018. https://whyy.org/articles/at-philly-zoo-louis-the-gorilla-takes-great-strides-to-round-up-snacks/.

Melore, Chris. 2022. "Humans May 'Evolve' to Have Deformed Bodies, Second Eyelid from Overusing Technology." Study Finds. November 2, 2022. https://studyfinds.org/humans-deformed-bodies-technology/.

O'Neil, Dennis. 2012. "Early Hominin Evolution: Discovery of Early Hominids." Palomar College. https://www.palomar.edu/anthro/hominid/australo_1.htm.

Ward, Peter. 2012. "What May Become of Homo Sapiens." *Scientific American* 22 (1s): 106–11. https://doi.org/10.1038/scientificamericanhuman1112-106.

CHAPTER 3: THE ANCIENT POSTURE

Bhishagratna, Kaviraj Kunja Lal. 1991. *An English Translation of the Sushruta Samhita: Based on Original Sanskrit Text: With a Full and Comprehensive Introduction, Additional Text, Different Readings, Notes, Comparative Views, Index, Glossary and Plates.* Varanasi: Chowkhamba Sanskrit Series Office.

Gugliotta, Guy. 2008. "The Great Human Migration." *Smithsonian Magazine.* July 1, 2008. https://www.smithsonianmag.com/history/the-great-human-migration-13561.

Nakou, Georgia. 2017. "Fitness Tips from Ancient Greece." Greece Is. January 6, 2017. https://www.greece-is.com/train-like-an-ancient-greek/.

O'Steen, Lisa, R. Ledbetter, and Daniel Elliott. 2017. "Archaic Period." *New Georgia Encyclopedia*, last modified Jun 6, 2017. https://www.georgiaencyclopedia.org/articles/history-archaeology/archaic-period-overview/

Tipton, Charles M. 2008. "Susruta of India, an Unrecognized Contributor to the History of Exercise Physiology." Journal of Applied Physiology 104 (6): 1553–56. https://doi.org/10.1152/japplphysiol.00925.2007

CHAPTER 4: 1,000 WAYS TO SIT

De Brito, Leonardo Barbosa Barreto, Djalma Rabelo Ricardo, Denise Sardinha Mendes Soares de Araújo, Plínio Santos Ramos, Jonathan Myers, and Claudio Gil Soares de Araújo. 2012. "Ability to Sit and Rise from the Floor as a Predictor of All-Cause Mortality." *European Journal of Preventive Cardiology* 21, no. 7: 892–98. https://doi.org/10.1177/2047487312471759.

Hewes, Gordon. 1957. "The Anthropology of Posture." *Scientific American*. February 1957. https://www.scientificamerican.com/article/the-anthropology-of-posture/.

International Association for the Study of Pain. 2021. "The Global Burden of Low Back Pain." International Association for the Study of Pain (IASP). 2021. https://www.iasp-pain.org/resources/fact-sheets/the-global-burden-of-low-back-pain/.

Kado, Deborah M., Mei-Hua Huang, Arun S. Karlamangla, Elizabeth Barrett-Connor, and Gail A. Greendale. 2004.

"Hyperkyphotic Posture Predicts Mortality in Older Community-Dwelling Men and Women: A Prospective Study." *Journal of the American Geriatrics Society* 52, no. 10: 1662–67. https://doi.org/10.1111/j.1532-5415.2004.52458.x.

Kaschube, Dorothea, and Duane Quiatt. 1998. "Gordon W. Hewes (1917–1997): Scholar, Scientist, General Anthropologist." *American Anthropologist* 100, no. 4: 984–87. https://doi.org/10.1525/aa.1998.100.4.984.

Raichlen, David A., Herman Pontzer, Theodore W. Zderic, Jacob A. Harris, Audax Z. P. Mabulla, Marc T. Hamilton, and Brian M. Wood. 2020. "Sitting, Squatting, and the Evolutionary Biology of Human Inactivity." *Proceedings of the National Academy of Sciences* 117, no. 13: 7115–21. https://doi.org/10.1073/pnas.1911868117.

Sohn, Emily. 2017. "How Does A Nepalese Porter Carry So Much Weight?" *NPR*, March 12, 2017. https://www.npr.org/sections/goatsandsoda/2017/03/12/517923490/how-does-a-nepalese-sherpa-carry-so-much-weight.

Volinn, Ernest. 1997. "The Epidemiology of Low Back Pain in the Rest of the World." *Spine* 22, no. 15: 1747–54. https://doi.org/10.1097/00007632-199708010-00013.

CHAPTER 5: IT STARTS YOUNG

Asimov, Nanette. 2003. "1 million Kids Fail Fitness Test / but State's Students Have Raised Scores." *SFGATE*, November 12, 2003. https://www.sfgate.com/health/article/1-million-kids-fail-fitness-test-But-state-s-2512363.php..

Candotti, Cláudia Tarragô, Silvia Elisandra B Nunes, Matias Noll, Kate de Freitas, and Carla Harzheim Macedo. 2011. "Efeitos de Um Programa de Educação Postural Para Crianças E Adolescentes Após Oito Meses de Seu Término." *Revista Paulista de Pediatria* 29, no. 4: 577–83. https://doi.org/10.1590/s0103-05822011000400017.

CDC Healthy Schools. 2021. "Physical Activity and Sedentary Behaviors and Academic Grades." February 1, 2021. https://www.cdc.gov/healthyschools/health_and_academics/physical-activity-and-sedentary-behaviors-and-academic-grades.htm.

Common Sense Media. 2011. "Screen usage from 0 to 8 years." https://www.ftc.gov/sites/default/files/documents/public_comments/california-00325%C2%A0/00325-82243.pdf.

David, Daniela, Cosimo Giannini, Francesco Chiarelli, and Angelika Mohn. 2021. "Text Neck Syndrome in Children and Adolescents." *International Journal of Environmental Research and Public Health* 18, no. 4: 1565. https://doi.org/10.3390/ijerph18041565.

Frampton, Roger. 2016. "Why Sitting down Destroys You | Roger Frampton | TEDxLeamingtonSpa." YouTube Video. https://www.youtube.com/watch?v=jOJLx4Du3vU.

Joyce, Michelle. 2017. *Posture Makeover: The Secret to Looking Great, Feeling Confident and Living Pain Free.* Eugene, OR: Posture Posse Press.

Kinnarps. N.d. "How Do You Create Good Ergonomics at School?" https://www.kinnarps.us/knowledge/how-do-you-create-good-ergonomics-at-school/.

National Physical Activity Plan Alliance. 2018. "The 2018 United States Report Card on Physical Activity for Children and Youth." https://paamovewithus.org/wp-content/uploads/2020/07/2018-US-Report-Card-PA-Children-Youth.pdf.

Chakravarty, Rupa. 2020. "Disturbing Trend – Poor Posture in Children -." Root Cause Medical Clinic. September 8, 2020. https://rootcausemedicalclinics.com/disturbing-trend-poor-posture-in-children/.

Tsukayama, Hayley. 2015. "Teens spend nearly nine hours every day consuming media." *Washington Post*, November 4, 2015. https://www.washingtonpost.com/news/the-switch/wp/2015/11/03/teens-spend-nearly-nine-hours-every-day-consuming-media/

CHAPTER 6: BREATHING SHAPES OUR BODY

Calais-Germain, Blandine. 2006. *Anatomy of Breathing*. Seattle, WA: Eastland Press.

Campbell, Thomas G, Tammy C Hoffmann, and Paul P Glasziou. 2018. "Buteyko Breathing for Asthma." *Cochrane Database of Systematic Reviews*, August 22, 2018. https://doi.org/10.1002/14651858.cd009158.pub2.

Goff, Sarah. 2022. "Asthma Facts | AAFA.Org." Asthma & Allergy Foundation of America. November 1, 2022. https://

aafa.org/asthma/asthma-facts/#:~:text=Approximately%20
25%20million%20Americans%20have,and%207%20
percent%20of%20children.

JMHI. 1995. "Diaphragm." *John Hopkins School of Medicine'
Interactive Respiratory Physiology Encyclopedia.* https://
oac.med.jhmi.edu/res_phys/Encyclopedia/Diaphragm/
Diaphragm.HTML.

Kang, Jeong-Il, Dae-Keun Jeong, and Hyun Choi. 2018.
"Correlation between Pulmonary Functions and
Respiratory Muscle Activity in Patients with Forward Head
Posture." *Journal of Physical Therapy Science* 30 (1): 132–35.
https://doi.org/10.1589/jpts.30.132.

Miller, Greg. 2022. "How Does Breathing Affect Your Brain?"
Smithsonian Magazine, October 18, 2022. https://www.
smithsonianmag.com/science-nature/how-does-breathing-
affect-your-brain-180980950/

Murphy, Jen. 2020. "The Need to Breathe." FLUX, September
21, 2020. https://fluxhawaii.com/freedive-hawaii-learn-to-
breathe/

Zeltner, Brie. 2010. "Buteyko—Institute of Breathing
and Health." Buteyko—Institute of Breathing and
Health. https://buteyko.info/.

CHAPTER 7: BREATHING SHAPES OUR BRAIN

Bond, Mary. 2006. *The New Rules of Posture.* New York, NY: Simon
and Schuster.

Bunch, Erin. 2021. "Box Breathing: How to Use the Technique to Combat Stress." Well+Good. April 4, 2021. https://www.wellandgood.com/box-breathing/.

Department of Health & Human Services. 2015. "Breathing to Reduce Stress." Better Health. https://www.betterhealth.vic.gov.au/health/healthyliving/breathing-to-reduce-stress.

Ma, Xiao, Zi-Qi Yue, Zhu-Qing Gong, Hong Zhang, Nai-Yue Duan, Yu-Tong Shi, Gao-Xia Wei, and You-Fa Li. 2017. "The Effect of Diaphragmatic Breathing on Attention, Negative Affect and Stress in Healthy Adults." *Frontiers in Psychology* 8, no. 874: 1–12. https://doi.org/10.3389/fpsyg.2017.00874.

Russo, Marc A., Danielle M. Santarelli, and Dean O'Rourke. 2017. "The Physiological Effects of Slow Breathing in the Healthy Human." *Breathe* 13, no. 4: 298–309. https://doi.org/10.1183/20734735.009817.

Wheeler, Kathryn. 2020. "Try the Breathing Technique That Improves Your Concentration." Happiful.com. August 6, 2020. https://happiful.com/try-the-breathing-technique-that-improves-your-concentration.

CHAPTER 8: RELAX

APA. 2013. "APA Survey Finds US Employers Unresponsive to Employee Needs." American Psychological Association, press release. https://www.apa.org/news/press/releases/2013/03/employee-needs.

Boyd, Danielle. 2019. "42 Worrying Workplace Stress Statistics."
The American Institute of Stress. September 23, 2019. https://
www.stress.org/42-worrying-workplace-stress-statistics.

Davis, Michelle. 2020. "Three Hours Longer, the Pandemic
Workday Has Obliterated Work-Life Balance." *Bloomberg*,
April 23, 2020. https://www.bloomberg.com/news/
articles/2020-04-23/working-from-home-in-covid-era-
means-three-more-hours-on-the-job#xj4y7vzkg.

Goldstein, David S. 2010. "Adrenal Responses to Stress." *Cellular
and Molecular Neurobiology* 30, no. 8: 1433–40. https://doi.
org/10.1007/s10571-010-9606-9.

Khazan, Inna. 2020. "Tech Stress: What It Is and How to
Prevent It. Conversation between Dr. Inna Khazan and Dr.
Erik Peper." YouTube Video. August 18, 2020. https://www.
youtube.com/watch?v=DzPnn0q6Aj8.

Peper, Erik. 2003. "The Integration of Electromyography
(SEMG) at the Workstation: Assessment, Treatment,
and Prevention of Repetitive Strain Injury." *Applied
Psychophysiology and Biofeedback* 28, no. 2: 167–82. https://
doi.org/10.1023/a:1023818810766.

CHAPTER 9: POSTURE FOR EMPOWERMENT

Briñol, Pablo, Richard E. Petty, and Benjamin Wagner. 2009.
"Body Posture Effects on Self-Evaluation: A Self-Validation
Approach." *European Journal of Social Psychology* 39, no. 6:
1053–64. https://doi.org/10.1002/ejsp.607.

Cuddy, Amy J. C., S. Jack Schultz, and Nathan E. Fosse. 2018. "P-Curving a More Comprehensive Body of Research on Postural Feedback Reveals Clear Evidential Value for Power-Posing Effects: Reply to Simmons and Simonsohn." *Psychological Science* 29, no. 4: 656–66. https://doi.org/10.1177/0956797617746749.

Ferry, Korn. 2018. "Worried Workers: Korn Ferry Survey Finds Professionals Are More Stressed out at Work Today than 5 Years Ago." November 8, 2018. https://www.kornferry.com/about-us/press/worried-workers-korn-ferry-survey-finds-professionals-are-more-stressed-out-at-work-today-than-5-years-ago.

First Up. "Employee App: 7 Reasons Why Your Company Needs One Today." June 24, 2022. https://firstup.io/blog/employee-app-seven-reasons-why-your-company-needs-one-today/.

Giang, Vivian. 2015. "The Surprising and Powerful Links between Posture and Mood." Fast Company. January 30, 2015. https://www.fastcompany.com/3041688/the-surprising-and-powerful-links-between-posture-and-mood

Hansen, Brianna. 2018. "Crash and Burnout: Is Workplace Stress the New Normal?" Wrike. https://www.wrike.com/blog/stress-epidemic-report-announcement/.

Holcroft, Rob. 2017. "Postural Empowerment: The Future of Holistic Wellbeing | Rob Holcroft | TEDxStoke." YouTube Video. March 18, 2017. https://www.youtube.com/watch?v=bKuDDNi5Dlw.

Nair, Shwetha, Mark Sagar, John Sollers, Nathan Consedine, and Elizabeth Broadbent. 2015. "Do Slumped and Upright Postures Affect Stress Responses? A Randomized Trial." *Health Psychology: Official Journal of the Division of Health Psychology, American Psychological Association* 34, no. 6: 632–41. https://doi.org/10.1037/hea0000146.

Ray, Julie. 2019. "Americans' Stress, Worry and Anger Intensified in 2018." Gallup. April 25, 2019. https://news.gallup.com/poll/249098/americans-stress-worry-anger-intensified-2018.aspx?utm_source=link_wwwv9&utm_campaign=item_248900&utm_medium=copy.

Spence, Jacq. 2020a. "Nonverbal Communication: How Body Language & Nonverbal Cues Are Key." Lifesize. February 18, 2020. https://www.lifesize.com/blog/speaking-without-words/.

Spring Health. 2022. "The Importance of Mental Health in the Workplace." March 1, 2022. https://springhealth.com/blog/importance-of-mental-health-workplace-wellness/.

Wilson, Vietta E., and Erik Peper. 2004. "The Effects of Upright and Slumped Postures on the Recall of Positive and Negative Thoughts." *Applied Psychophysiology and Biofeedback* 29, no. 3: 189–95. https://doi.org/10.1023/b:apbi.0000039057.32963.34.

CHAPTER 10: ACTIVITY—THE ANTIDOTE TO THE SITTING DISEASE

Bowman, Katy Ann. 2014. Move Your DNA: *Restore Your Health through Natural Movement*. Carlsborg, WA: Propriometrics Press.

Church, Timothy S., Diana M. Thomas, Catrine Tudor-Locke, Peter T. Katzmarzyk, Conrad P. Earnest, Ruben Q. Rodarte, Corby K. Martin, Steven N. Blair, and Claude Bouchard. 2011. "Trends over 5 Decades in U.S. Occupation-Related Physical Activity and Their Associations with Obesity." Edited by Alejandro Lucia. *PLoS ONE* 6, no. 5: e19657. https://doi.org/10.1371/journal.pone.0019657.

Curtin, Sally C. 2019. "Trends in Cancer and Heart Disease Death Rates Among Adults Aged 45-64: United States, 1999-2017." *National vital statistics reports: from the Centers for Disease Control and Prevention, National Center for Health Statistics, National Vital Statistics System* 68, no. 5: 1–9. https://pubmed.ncbi.nlm.nih.gov/32501204/.

Davis, Nicola. 2019. "Sit Less and Move More to Reduce Risk of Early Death, Study Says." *The Guardian*, January 14, 2019. https://www.theguardian.com/society/2019/jan/14/sit-less-and-move-more-to-reduce-risk-of-early-death-study-says.

Edwardson, Charlotte L, Tom Yates, Stuart J H Biddle, Melanie J Davies, David W Dunstan, Dale W Esliger, Laura J Gray, et al. 2018. "Effectiveness of the Stand More at (SMArT) Work Intervention: Cluster Randomised Controlled Trial." *The BMJ* 363 (October 10): k3870. https://doi.org/10.1136/bmj.k3870.

Fiorenzi, Ryan. 2018. "Start Standing." Start Standing. April 3, 2018. https://www.startstanding.org/sitting-new-smoking/.

Nazario, Brunilda. 2021. "Surprising Causes of High Cholesterol." WebMD. https://www.webmd.com/cholesterol-management/ss/slideshow-surprising-causes-high-cholesterol.

Maxwell, Gill. 2008. "Case Study Series on Work-Life Balance in Large Organizations." Society for Human Resource Management. https://www.shrm.org/certification/educators/Documents/Worklife%20Balance%20Case%20Final_SW.pdf.

Saeidifard, Farzane, Jose R Medina-Inojosa, Marta Supervia, Thomas P Olson, Virend K Somers, Patricia J Erwin, and Francisco Lopez-Jimenez. 2018. "Differences of Energy Expenditure While Sitting versus Standing: A Systematic Review and Meta-Analysis." *European Journal of Preventive Cardiology* 25, no. 5: 522–38. https://doi.org/10.1177/2047487317752186

Schulte, Brigid. 2015. "Health Experts Have Figured out How Much Time You Should Sit Each Day." *Chicago Tribune.* June 3, 2015. https://www.chicagotribune.com/lifestyles/health/ct-dangers-of-sitting-20150601-story.html.

Scutti, Susan. 2017. "Yes, Sitting Too Long Can Kill You, Even If You Exercise." *CNN*, September 11, 2017. https://www.cnn.com/2017/09/11/health/sitting-increases-risk-of-death-study/index.html.

Smith, Jonathon A. B., Mladen Savikj, Parneet Sethi, Simon Platt, Brendan M. Gabriel, John A. Hawley, David Dunstan, Anna Krook, Juleen R. Zierath, and Erik Näslund. 2021. "Three weeks of interrupting sitting lowers fasting glucose and glycemic variability, but not glucose tolerance, in free-living women and men with obesity." *American Journal of Physiology–Endocrinology and Metabolism* 321, no. 2: E203-E216. https://journals.physiology.org/doi/full/10.1152/ajpendo.00599.2020.

Williams, Jason. 2021. "Why Do I Have Low Back Pain While Sitting?" Access Health Chiropractic. July 8, 2021. https://www.accesshealthchiro.com/why-do-i-have-low-back-pain-while-sitting/.

World Health Organization. 2022. "Indicator Metadata Registry Details." WHO. https://www.who.int/data/gho/indicator-metadata-registry/imr-details/3416.

CHAPTER 11: SYMMETRY MATTERS

Lu, Tung-Wu, and Chu-Fen Chang. "Biomechanics of Human Movement and Its Clinical Applications." *The Kaohsiung Journal of Medical Sciences* 28, no. 2 (February): S13–S25, www.sciencedirect.com/science/article/pii/S1607551X11001835.

Comerford, M.J., and S.L. Mottram. 2001. "Movement and Stability Dysfunction—Contemporary Developments." *Manual Therapy* 6, no. 1: 15–26. https://doi.org/10.1054/math.2000.0388.

Moore, Rebecca. 2020. "The Janda Approach to Chronic Pain Syndromes." Performance Health Academy. https://www.performancehealthacademy.com/the-janda-approach-to-chronic-pain-syndromes.html.

Joseph J. Knapik et al., "Strength, Flexibility and Athletic Injuries1," *Sports Medicine* 14, no. 5 (November): 277–88, https://doi.org/10.2165/00007256-199214050-00001.

Smidt, Gary L. 1994. "Current Open and Closed Kinetic Chain Concepts—Clarifying or Confusing?" *Journal of Orthopaedic & Sports Physical Therapy* 20, no. 5: 235–35. https://doi.org/10.2519/jospt.1994.20.5.235.

Physiopedia. 2023. "Single Leg Stance Test." https://www.physiopedia.com/Single_Leg_Stance_Test.

Araujo, Claudio Gil, Christina Grüne de Souza e Silva, Jari Antero Laukkanen, Maria Fiatarone Singh, Setor Kunutsor, Jonathan Myers, João Felipe Franca, and Claudia Lucia Castro. 2022. "Successful 10-Second One-Legged Stance Performance Predicts Survival in Middle-Aged and Older Individuals." *British Journal of Sports Medicine* 56, no. 17: 975–980. https://doi.org/10.1136/bjsports-2021-105360.

Mosley, Michael. 2022. "Dr Michael Mosley: Take the Balance Challenge to Help You Live Longer." *BBC Science Focus Magazine.* March 2022. https://www.sciencefocus.com/the-human-body/dr-michael-mosley-standing-on-one-leg/.

CHAPTER 12: IPOSTURE

Eidelson, Stewart G. 2019. "Cervical Spine Anatomy (Neck)." SpineUniverse. https://www.spineuniverse.com/anatomy/cervical-spine-anatomy-neck.

Gekhman, Dmitriy. "Mass of a Human Head." The Physics Factbook website. Edited by Glenn Elert. https://hypertextbook.com/facts/2006/DmitriyGekhman.shtml.

Hansraj, Kenneth K. "Assessment of stresses in the cervical spine caused by posture and position of the head." *Surgical Technology International* 11, no. 25: 277–279. https://pubmed.ncbi.nlm.nih.gov/25393825/.

Hesiod. 1997. *Theogony*. Translated by M L West. Oxford; New York: Clarendon Press.

Middlesworth, Matt. 2015. "A Six-Point Checklist to Correctly Position Your Computer Monitor." ErgoPlus. August 7, 2015. https://ergo-plus.com/office-ergonomics-position-computer-monitor/.

TEDx Talks. 2018. "Posture: The Key to Good Health | Annette Verpillot | TEDxMontrealWomen." YouTube Video. https://www.youtube.com/watch?v=S3qdSo8zoIs.

CHAPTER 13: AT THE CENTER OF IT

Al-Eisa, Einas, David Egan, and Anne Fenety. 2004. "Association between Lateral Pelvic Tilt and Asymmetry in Sitting Pressure Distribution." *Journal of Manual & Manipulative Therapy* 12, no. 3: 133–42. https://doi.org/10.1179/106698104790825239.

Barr, Karen P., Miriam Griggs, and Todd Cadby. 2005. "Lumbar Stabilization." *American Journal of Physical Medicine &*

Rehabilitation 84, no. 6: 473–80. https://doi.org/10.1097/01.
phm.0000163709.70471.42.

Ko, Kwang-Jun, et al., "Effects of 12-Week Lumbar Stabilization
Exercise and Sling Exercise on Lumbosacral Region Angle,
Lumbar Muscle Strength, and Pain Scale of Patients with
Chronic Low Back Pain," *Journal of Physical Therapy Science*
30, no. 1 (January): 18–22, https://doi.org/10.1589/jpts.30.18.

Poli, Angelo. 2013. "Realigned—Technology's Impact on
Our Posture | Angelo Poli | TEDxChico." YouTube
Video. December 4, 2013. https://www.youtube.com/
watch?v=BxuqmF1GbxU.

Porterfield, James A., and Carl DeRosa, *Mechanical Low Back
Pain: Perspectives in Functional Anatomy*. Philadelphia, PA:
Saunders.

Starrett, Kelly. 2016. *Deskbound: Sitting Is the New Smoking*.
Cleveland, OH: Victory Belt Publishing.

Takaki, Sho, Koji Kaneoka, Yu Okubo, Satoru Otsuka, Masaki
Tatsumura, Itsuo Shiina, and Shumpei Miyakawa. "Analysis
of Muscle Activity during Active Pelvic Tilting in Sagittal
Plane." *Physical Therapy Research* 19, no. 1: 50–57. https://doi.
org/10.1298/ptr.e9900.

CHAPTER 14: WALK THIS WAY

Book, Angela, Kimberly Costello, and Joseph A. Camilleri.
2013. "Psychopathy and Victim Selection." *Journal of*

Interpersonal Violence 28, no. 11: 2368–83. https://doi.
org/10.1177/0886260512475315.

Dimon, Theodore, and John Qualter. 2008. *Anatomy of the
Moving Body: A Basic Course in Bones, Muscles, and Joints.*
Berkeley, CA.: North Atlantic Books.

Johnson, Paul. n.d. "Over Pronation Explained." Manchester
Sports Podiatry and Gait Clinic. Accessed February 20,
2023. https://manchestersportspodiatry.co.uk/pronation-
explained/.

Nguyen, Uyen-Sa D T, et al. 2011. "Increasing prevalence of
knee pain and symptomatic knee osteoarthritis: survey and
cohort data." *Annals of Internal Medicine* 155, no. 11: 725–32.
https://doi:10.7326/0003-4819-155-11-201112060-00004.

Sánchez-Rodríguez, Raquel, Alfonso Martínez-Nova, Elena
Escamilla-Martínez, and Juan Diego Pedrera-Zamorano.
2012. "Can the Foot Posture Index or Their Individual
Criteria Predict Dynamic Plantar Pressures?" *Gait & Posture*
36, no. 3: 591–95. https://doi.org/10.1016/j.gaitpost.2012.05.024.

Schrupp, Bob, and Brad Heineck. 2016. "Knock Knees? Causes
and Results. What Causes Your Knees to 'Go In'?" YouTube
Video. https://www.youtube.com/watch?v=ZWh1hTYjirE.

Sivacolundhu, Suresh. 2018. "Foot Pronation: Underpronation
& Overpronation Explained." The Foot Clinic. February 4,
2018. https://thefootclinic.net/foot-pronation-podiatrist-
cottesloe-perth/.

Printed in Great Britain
by Amazon